Hyperlipidaemia - Ayurvedic Principles and Treatments

An Effective Treatment Based on Holistic Approach and Clinical Study

Hyperlipidaemia - Ayurvedic Principles and Treatments

An Effective Treatment Based on Holistic Approach and Clinical Study

Khyati Rohit

ELIVA PRESS

ISBN: 978-99949-8-724-5

Cover Design: Eliva Press
Cover Image: Ingimage
Email: info@elivapress.com
Website: www.elivapress.com

This Eliva Press imprint is published by the registered company Eliva Press Global Ltd. part of Eliva Press S.R.L. Publishing Group

The registered company address is: Pope Hennessy Street Level 2, Hennessy Tower Port Louis, Mauritius
Eliva Press S.R.L. Publishing Group address is: Bulevardul Moscova 21, Chisinau, Moldova, Europe

HYPERLIPIDAEMIA - AYURVEDIC PRINCIPLES AND TREATMENTS

An Effective Treatment Based On Holistic Approach And Clinical Study

AUTHOR – DR. KHYATI ROHIT

BAMS MD(Ayu.Medicine)PGDEMS

Consulting Ayurveda Physician

Mumbai, India

ABSTRACT:

Hyperlipidaemia is one such lifestyle disorder which is identified as an impending risk factor for many diseases like hypertension, metabolic syndrome, coronary artery disease (CAD) and cerebrovascular diseases (CVD). In Hyperlipidaemia levels of lipoproteins i.e. (cholesterol, triglycerides, or both) are raised in the plasma, which can be co-related to elevated Sneha(Oil) or Meda Dhatu(Fatty tissue) in the body. As drugs used in modern medicine viz. statins, fibrates etc. to treat hyperlipidaemia has several adverse effects such as myopathy, potential elevation in serum transaminase levels leading to hepatic damage, nausea or vomiting, bowel upset, multiple joint pain etc. Hence, it is very much necessary to have definite and harmless solution to this problem. There is a major role of Agni(Metabolic fire) and Ama(Undigested/unripedsubstance) in pathogenesis of hyperlipidaemia, and the drugs having Dipana(Augmenting), Pachana(Digestive), Ama Nasahak(Destroyer of undigested food), Kaphamedohara(Mitigating phlegm and fat),Srotoshodhak(Purification of channels) , Rasayan (Rejuvenator) quality will be highly effective for the management of hyperlipidaemia. Apatarpan(Undernutrition) is the treatment advocated in ayurved for Santarpanjanya Vyadhis(Diseases of overnutrition) and Hyperlipidaemia is one among this group of disease. Taking into consideration all the treatment modalities in Ayurveda, Rasarakta Pachak Ghanavati was given as a line of treatment in Hyperlipidaemia. Methods - 60 patients of Hyperlipidaemia as per the objective criteria of range for lipid profile mentioned in American Journal of Lifestyle Medicine were randomly selected from OPD and IPD of Dr. D. Y. Patil College of Ayurved and Research centre, Pimpri, Pune,India.Group A (n=30) patients were treated with Rasarakta Pachak Ghanavati (500mg) 2 tabs twice in a day after food for 30 days and Group B (n=30) patients were treated with Tab Atorvastatin (10mg) 1 tab once in a day after food for 30 days.

Result- Rasarakta Pachak Ghanavati group showed marked improvement on Serum Total Cholesterol and Serum LDL – Cholesterol and moderate improvement on Serum Triglycerides and Serum HDL – Cholesterol parameters of lipid profile. While Tab Atorvastatin group showed marked improvement on almost all the parameters of lipid profile.

KEYWORDS: Hyperlipidaemia, Meda dhatu, Ama, Agni, Rasarakta pachak ghanavati, Apatarpan chikitsa, Lipid profile, Cholesterol.

CONTENTS

CHAPTER 1 - INTRODUCTION

21st century is the century of science and technology. Newer discoveries of the science have made human life very fast and easy. Physical work is replaced by mental work. With the help of science man is climbing the steps of success, but moving away from nature. This condition has given birth to various Lifestyle diseases.

As a result of the growing challenges of modernization, man has responded by readapting his habitual behaviour. Man has adapted himself to the fast paced life by modifying his dietary and lifestyle preferences to suit the modern era. This has resulted in a state of inconsistency between the external environment and his internal mechanism causing multitudes of diseases which are popularly are referred as lifestyle diseases.

The human life is rapidly changing in its food, standard of living, environment, profession, etc. Because of sedentary standard of living and drastic changes in food pattern a major fraction of human population is suffering from disorders like Coronary artery diseases, Diabetes mellitus, Atherosclerosis, Cerebrovascular accident etc.

Fast foods, lack of exercise, irregular sleep, stress, various addictions etc. are some of the factors which contribute greatly to such diseases. These factors generally act by impairing the metabolism of an individual making him prone to series of disorders. Hyperlipidaemia is one such disorder which is identified as a potential risk factor for multitudes of diseases like cardiovascular diseases, metabolic syndrome and even hypertension. Hyperlipidaemia and Hypertension are two risk factors that commonly co- exist and are modifiable through medications and or lifestyle changes.

Hyperlipidaemia is one of the most important contributing factors to the atherosclerosis of large and medium sized arteries, leading to coronary Heart disease (CHD). Cardiovascular diseases (CVDs) are the most prevalent cause of death in both developed as well as developing countries. Rapid urbanization and its accompanying adverse lifestyle changes are likely to be the risk factors of Cardio vascular diseases.

The term hyperlipidaemia signifies an elevation of lipid or fat content in the blood. “Hyper” means high, “lipid” is another word for fat or fat like substance, “emia” refers to the blood. It is an abnormal amount of lipids (cholesterol or fat) in the blood. Hyperlipidaemia or hyperlipoproteinaemia is the condition of abnormally elevated levels of any or all lipids and or lipoproteins in the blood. It is the most common form of dyslipidaemia (which also includes any decreased lipid levels).

Hyperlipidaemia is relatively silent as far as what patient can notice on his or her own. Hence, it is a silent killer. It is a condition in which the levels of lipoproteins i.e. (cholesterol, triglycerides or both) are raised in the plasma; which can be co-related to raised 'Meda' (Fat) in the body.

Although the texts of Ayurveda do not directly describe the terms like hyperlipidaemia, but sufficient descriptions are scattered throughout the Ayurvedic Samhitas (texts). The lipids, which are described in modern science, have properties which closely bear a resemblance with the properties of "Sneha Dravya" (Unctuous substance). Meda (fatty tissue), Vasa (fatty deposits) and Majja (bone marrow) can be correlated with the lipids on the basis of their properties. As long as they are within their normal physiological state they are considered as "Dhatu"(tissue) and "Upadhatu"(subtissue) because they constitute our body. Any increase in their levels in the body is considered as pathological, as these factors are capable of producing various lipid disorders in our body. Medo Dushti (Vitiation of fatty tissue) as described in Ayurvedic texts resembles with the disorder of modern medicine termed as hyperlipidaemia.

Attempts were made by various scholars of Ayurveda to clinically co – relate it to Rasagat Sneha Vriddhi (increase of unctuousness in plasma), Raktagat Sneha Vriddhi (increase of unctuousness in blood), Rasaraktagat Sneha Vriddhi (increase of unctuousness in plasma & blood), Medoroga (diseases of fat), Medo Vriddhi (increase in fat), Ama Medo Dhatu (undigested fatty tissue), Sthaulya (obesity), etc. A detailed study of hyperlipidaemia reveals its similarity to Asthayi Medo Dhatu Vriddhi (Increase of unstable fatty tissue) on the basis of its pathophysiology. Also this excessively increased Asthayi Medo Dhatu (unstable fatty tissue) is Ama (undigested/unriped substance) in nature due to which it is retained in the body for a longer time resulting in further complications.

By considering all the situations it can be presumed that the pathology is related to Kapha Karaka Nidana (phlegm forming cause) i.e. – Santarpana Ahara & vihara (overnutritious dietetics & daily regime) , which includes sedentary life style, high calories food intake , lack of exercise,etc which finally leads to morbidity of Kapha Dosha (phlegm) and Medo Dhatu (fatty tissue). Due to Medodhatvagnimandya (impairement in metabolic tissue fire of fatty tissue) and Dushti (vitiation) excessive accumulation of abnormal Kapha (phlegm) and Meda (fat) occurs in various Srotas (channels) in body. Aparipakva Kapha – Meda (unriped/ immature phlegm-fat) present in Rasa- Raktavaha Srotas (channels of plasma & blood) results in obstruction to the movement of Vata (air) and Rakta (blood) through affected channels, which finally ends up in disease manifestation according to the site of disease. The state of Apakva Kapha (unriped phlegm) or Meda (fat) and its excessive presence, Margavaran (obstruction of path) in Rasa- Raktavaha Srotas (channels of plasma & blood) is often compared with the state of Dyslipidaemia

CHAPTER 2- MODERN REVIEW OF LIPIDS

2.1 – Introduction Of Lipids :

The term 'lipid' refers to substance with poor water solubility. Biologically important lipids include sterols, which are composed of hydrocarbon rings, and glycerides (including triglycerides and phospholipids), which are chiefly composed of hydrocarbon chains (including fatty acids). Lipids constitute a heterogeneous group of compounds, which are relatively insoluble in water, but freely soluble in non-polar organic solvents like benzene, chloroform, ether, acetone, etc. They are of great importance to the body as the chief concentrated storage forms of energy, besides their role in cellular structure and various other biochemical functions.

Etymology: - [lip'id , li'pid]

Greek word – lipos, fat, eidos, are of great importance to the body as the chief concentrated storage form of energy.

Lipids are nonpolar hydrophobic molecules comprising the essential components of all living cells. In the human body they perform several important functions by playing an important role in the cellular structure, serving as concentrated storage forms of energy, metabolic regulators, protecting internal organs by a cushioning effect etc. Some of these lipids, stored in the body areas are known as depot lipids where as others circulate in the blood.

The lipids present in the body physiologically form two components:

1. **Element Constant or structural lipids –** Cytoplasma and cell membrane of all organs are composed of element constant, so that their fat content does not diminish in starvation. The value of this lipid remains constant. It is present in the body in fixed proportions and constitutes structural components of the body like phospholipids and thus it is essential for life.
2. **Element Variable –** It is present in variable amounts and serves to nourish other body structures like neutral fat. It is chiefly composed of neutral fat. It is present mostly in the depot fat or adipose tissue in free form and represents stored energy.

2.2 Classification of Lipids :

1. Simple Lipids –

These are esters of fatty acids with alcohols.

a) Neutral fats: Triglycerides, Esters of various fatty acids with glycerol.

b) Waxes: Cholesterol and its esters.

2. Compound Lipids –

These are esters of fatty acids with alcohols containing additional groups such as phosphate, nitrogenous base, carbohydrate, protein, etc. They are further divided as follow:

a) Phospholipids: They contain phosphoric acid and a nitrogenous base i.e. lecithin, cephalin.

b) Glycolipids: Esters containing a carbohydrate and a nitrogenous base i.e. - cerebrosides.

c) Sulpholipids : Esters containing sulphuric acid

d) Lipoproteins: Macromolecular ccomplexes of lipids with proteins.

3. Derived Lipids –

These are Derivatives obtained on the hydrolysis of group 1 and group 2 lipids which possess the characteristics of lipids. This includes glycerol and other alcohols, fatty acids, lipid soluble vitamins, steroid hormones, hydrogen carbons.

2.3 Depot Fats:

Fat in the body is present in two forms i.e. Plasma Lipids and Depot fat. About 12% of the total body weight of a man consists of fat. The major part of it remains stored. This is known as Depot fats.

Distribution of fat in body tissue:

i) Subcutaneous tissue – 50%

ii) Peripheral tissue – 15%

iii) Mesentery – 20%

iv) Omentum – 10%

v) Intramuscular connective tissue – 05%

Composition of depot fats:

Depot fat is mainly composed of mixed triglycerides. Trace of lecithin and cholesterol, as well as a little amount of polyunsaturated fatty acids.

Sources of depot fat:

The depot fat may be derived from:

1. Food fat: This is the main source.
2. Carbohydrates
3. Proteins

Functions of depot fat:

1. Mechanical – Depot fat provides protection against injury.
2. Physical – Regulation of body temperature.
3. Chemical – Storage of energy.

2.4 Plasma Lipids:

There are four main categories of lipids present in plasma in varying amount.

1. Cholesterol and its esters.
2. Triglycerides.
3. Phospholipids.
4. Non- esterified fatty acids (NEFA).

As lipids are present in both body cell and plasma of blood, but the composition of lipids in plasma and cells vary widely.Since the composition of plasma lipids accurately reflects the actual state of lipid metabolism, so the composition of plasma lipids is generally studied.

The composition of blood lipids is not a static because of process of addition and removal of lipids from blood:

Addition of lipids takes place by following ways:

1. Absorption from intestine
2. Synthesis of fat and its mobilization

Removal of lipids takes place in following ways:

1. Deposition of fat in the depot structures.
2. Oxidation of fat in the tissue.
3. Utilization for formation of tissue components.

1. Cholesterol And Its Esters :

Cholesterol is an organic chemical substance classified as a waxy steroid of fat. It is the most important animal steroid which forms an important structural component of cell membrane and is required to establish proper membrane permeability and fluidity. It is widely distributed in all the cells and is a major component of cell membranes and lipoproteins. Cholesterol is also an important component for the manufacture of bile acids, steroid hormones and vitamin D. About 70% of the cholesterol in the lipoproteins of the plasma is in the form of cholesterol esters. Cholesterol is synthesized in most of the body tissue of the body except Central Nervous System (Wilson, 1968).

Functions:

1. It is a structural component of cell membrane.
2. Cholesterol is required to build and maintain membranes; it regulates membrane fluidity over the range of physiological temperatures.
3. It helps to insulate nerve fibres, being a poor conductor of electricity.
4. It is the precursor for the synthesis of all other steroids in the body. These includes steroid hormones, vitamin D and bile acids. It is a precursor of bile which is essential for fat absorption.
5. It prevents toxins from entering into the cells.
6. It is an essential ingredient in the structure of lipoproteins in which form the lipids in the body are transported.

The clinical significance of cholesterol lies in the fact that recent studies have related increased levels of plasma cholesterol to the development of atherosclerosis which may further lead to cerebrovascular accidents or coronary artery diseases.

Dietary sources:

Animal fats are complex mixtures of triglycerides, with lesser amounts of phospholipids and cholesterol. As a consequence, all foods containing animal fat contain cholesterol to varying extent. Major dietary sources of cholesterol include cheese, egg yolks, beef, pork, and poultry. Human breast milk also contains significant quantities of cholesterol. Cholesterol is not present in plant based food sources unless it has been added during the food's preparation. However, plant products such as flax seeds and peanuts contain cholesterol like compounds called phytosterols, which are suggested to help lower serum cholesterol levels.

Saturated fat is present in full fat dairy products, animal fats, and several types of oil and chocolate. Tran's fats are typically derived from the partial hydrogenation of unsaturated fats. Tran's fat is most often encountered in margarine and hydrogenated vegetable fat, and consequently in many fast foods, snack foods, and fried baked foods.

Formation of cholesterol:

Besides the cholesterol absorbed each day from the gastrointestinal tract, which is called exogenous cholesterol, an even greater quantity is formed in the cells of the body called endogenous cholesterol. Essentially all the endogenous cholesterol that circulates in the lipoproteins of the plasma is formed by the liver, but all other cells of the body form at least some cholesterol, which is consistent with the fact that many of the membranous structures of all cells are partially composed of this substance. About 20-25% of total daily cholesterol production occurs in the liver; other sites of higher synthesis rates include the intestines, adrenal glands, and reproductive organs. The basic structure of cholesterol is a sterol nucleus. This is synthesized entirely from molecules of acetyl-CoA. In turn, the sterol nucleus can be modified by means of various side chains to form (1) cholesterol; (2) cholic acid, which is the basis of the bile acids, formed in the liver; and (3) many important steroid hormones secreted by the adrenal cortex, the ovaries, and the testes.

Synthesis and intake:

Cholesterol is derived in the human body via two sources: dietary sources (exogenous) or synthesized within the body (endogenous) production in which it is primarily synthesized from acetyl CoA through HMG – CoA reductase pathway. An average diet provides about 300mg of cholesterol per day whereas the body synthesizes about 700mg of cholesterol per day. About 20-25% of total daily production (~1/day) occurs in the liver; other sites of higher synthesis rates include the intestines, adrenal glands and reproductive organs. Now it is known that all nucleated cells can synthesize cholesterol including arterial walls. Cholesterol is absent in plants hence a vegetarian gets all his required cholesterol in the body from endogenous synthesis.

Regulation:

Biosynthesis of cholesterol is directly regulated by the cholesterol Levels present through the homeostatic mechanisms involved are only partly understood. A higher intake in food leads to a net decrease in endogenous production and vice versa. The main regulatory mechanism is the sensing of intracellular cholesterol in the endoplasmic reticulum by the proteins SREBP (Sterol Regulatory Element Binding Protein 1 and 2). SREBP (Sterol Regulatory Element Binding Protein) cuts on the falling of cholesterol levels and then migrates to the nucleus and acts as a transcription factor to bind to the "Sterol Regulatory Element

Catabolism:

Liver is the main site of cholesterol catabolism. Out of the daily production of 1000 mg of cholesterol, about 50% of cholesterol of liver is converted to bile acids and excreted in bile. Of this a part is reabsorbed from intestines whereas the unabsorbed portion is acted upon by the intestinal bacteria to form cholestanol and coprostanol (faecal sterols), this coprostanol is excreted in faeces along with the bile salts. The remaining 50% of cholesterol is converted into bile acids, which are excreted in the bile as bile salts.

Transport of cholesterol:

Cholesterol is only slightly soluble in water; it can dissolve and travel in the water based bloodstream at excedingly small concentrations. Since cholesterol is insoluble in blood, it is transported in the circulatory system within lipoproteins, complex spherical particles which have an exterior composed of amphiphilic proteins and lipids whose outward facing surfaces are water soluble and inward facing surfaces are lipid soluble; triglycerides and cholesterol esters are carried internally. Phospholipids and cholesterol, being amphipathic, are transported in the surface monolayer of the lipoprotein particle.

Metabolism, recycling and excretion:

Cholesterol is oxidized by the liver into a variety of bile acids. These in turn are conjugated with glycine, taurine, glucuronic acid or sulphate. A mixture of conjugated and non-conjugated bile acids along with cholesterol itself is excreted from liver into the bile. Approximately 95% of the bile acids are reabsorbed from the intestines and the remainder lost in the faeces. The excretion and reabsorption of bile acids forms the basis of the enterohepatic circulation which is essential for the digestion and absorption of dietary fats.

2. Triglycerides :

Triglycerides, also known as triacyl glycerol or neutral fats which are esters of glycerol and fatty acids. They are insoluble in water and nonpolar in character. It can be derived from both exogenously and endogenously.

The exogenous Triglyceride is derived from diet and it circulates in the blood in the form of chylomicrons. The endogenous form is synthesized in the liver. Liver and adipose tissue are the major sites of triglycerides synthesis.

The triglycerides constitute 95% of the adipose tissue, where they are mainly used for the storage of energy whereas in the liver triglycerides are mainly secreted as a very low density lipoprotein (VLDL). These triglycerides are broken down to free fatty acids and utilized as an energy source. It is an ester composed of glycerol bound to three fatty acids. It is the main constituent of vegetable oil and animal fats.

Metabolism:

The enzyme pancreatic lipase acts at the ester bond, hydrolysing the bond and releasing the fatty acid. In triglyceride form, lipids cannot be absorbed by the duodenum. Fatty acids, monoglycerides (one glycerol, one glycerol) and some diglycerides are absorbed by the duodenum, once the triglycerides have been broken down.

Triglycerides, as a major components of very low density lipoprotein (VLDL) and chylomicrons plays an important role in metabolism energy sources and transporters of dietary fat. In the intestine, triglycerides are split into monoacylglycerol and free fatty acids in a process called lipolysis, with the secretion of lipase and bile, which are subsequently moved to absorptive enterocytes from their fragments and packed together with cholesterol and proteins to form chylomicrons. These are excreted from the cells and collected by the lymph system and transported to the large vessels near the heart before being mixed into the blood. Various tissues can capture the chylomicrons, releasing the triglycerides to be used as a source of energy. Fat and liver cells can synthesize and store triglycerides. When the body requires fatty acids as an energy source, the hormone glucagon signals the breakdown of the triglycerides by hormone – sensitive lipase to release free fatty acids.Triglycerides cannot pass through cell membranes freely. Special enzymes on the walls of blood vessels called lipoprotein lipases must break down triglycerides into free fatty acids and glycerol. Then fatty acids can be taken up by cells via the fatty acid transporter (FAT).

3. Phospholipids :

Phospholipids are conjugated lipids which contain glycerol, fatty acids and a nitrogen base. These are complex or compound lipids containing phosphoric acid. The main plasma phospholipids are lecithin, sphingomyelin and the cephalins. They constitute about 25% LDL (Low density lipoprotein) and 30% HDL (High density lipoprotein).

Uses:

- Phospholipids are essential for the synthesis of different lipoproteins
- They participate in the absorption of fat from the intestine.
- Phospholipids participate in the reverse cholesterol transport and thus help in the removal of cholesterol from the body.

4. Non – Esterified Fatty Acids (NEFA):

Also termed as free fatty acids, they are complexed with albumin in the plasma and mainly derived from the lipolysis of triglycerides stored in the adipose tissue. They are important sources of energy. They function either to supply energy by oxidation or are incorporated into tissue lipids by esterification.

2.5 Lipoproteins:

Lipoproteins are molecular complexes that contains both proteins and lipids (conjugated proteins) cells. Lipoproteins are the small particles in the blood which contain cholesterol, phospholipids, triglycerides and proteins. They are transport vehicles for lipids in the circulation. Many enzymes, transporters, structural proteins, antigens, adhesins, and toxins are lipoproteins. Examples include the high- density lipoproteins (HDL) and low- density lipoproteins (LDL), which enable fats to be carried in the blood stream, the transmembrane proteins of the mitochondrion and the chloroplast, and bacterial lipoproteins.

Lipoproteins are large mostly spherical complexes of lipids and proteins that transport lipids (primarily triglycerides, cholesterol esters, and fat soluble vitamins) through the body fluids (plasma, interstitial fluid and lymph). Their functions are:

1. In the absorption of dietary cholesterol, long chain fatty acids, and fat-soluble vitamins.
2. The transport of triglycerides, cholesterol, and fat soluble vitamins from the liver to the peripheral tissues;
3. The transport of cholesterol from the peripheral tissues to the liver.

Depending upon density the lipoproteins in plasma are classified into 5 major categories:

1. Chylomicrons – It carries triglycerides from the intestine to liver, skeletal muscle, and to adipose tissue.
2. Very low density lipoproteins (VLDL) or pre- beta lipoproteins – It carries (newly synthesized) triacylglycerol from the liver to adipose tissue. It contains high concentration of triglycerides (formed from FFA and glycerol) and moderate concentration of cholesterol and phospholipids.
3. Intermediate density lipoproteins (IDL) or broad- beta lipoproteins- are intermediate between VLDL and LDL. They are not usually detectable in the blood. Formed by the removal of large portion of triglycerides from VLDL by lipoprotein lipase.
4. Low density lipoproteins (LDL) or beta lipoproteins- It carries cholesterol from the liver to cells of the body. Formed from IDL by the complete removal of triglycerides. These lipoproteins contain only cholesterol and phospholipids. LDL's are sometimes referred to as the "bad cholesterol" lipoprotein.

5. High density lipoproteins (HDL) or alpha lipoproteins – It collects cholesterol from the body's tissues, and bring it back to the liver. It contains high concentrations of proteins with low concentration of cholesterol and phospholipids. HDLs are sometimes referred to as the "Good cholesterol" lipoprotein.

Table No 1: Characteristics of different classes of lipoproteins:

Composition	**Chylomicrons**	**VLDL(Very Low density lipoprotein)**	**LDL (Low density lipoprotein)**	**HDL (High density lipoprotein)**
Protein %	1-2	7-10	18-22	45-55
Lipid %	99	93	80	50
Major lipid	Triglyceride	Triglyceride	Cholesterol	Cholesterol phospholipids
Diameter(nm)	80-500	30-100	21.5	7.5-10.5
Origin	Intestine	Liver and intestine	End product of VLDL	Liver and intestine
Function	Transport Exogenous Triglyceride	Transport Exogenous Triglyceride	Transport of cholesterol & phospholipids to peripheral cells	Proposed to transport cholesterol from peripheral cells to liver

Table no : 2 Functions of Lipoproteins:

Primary function of lipoproteins is to transport the lipids via blood to and from the tissues.

Lipoproteins	**Functions**
VLDL (Very Low density lipoprotein)	Transports triglycerides from liver to adipose tissue.
IDL (Intermediate density lipoprotein)	Transports triglycerides, cholesterol and phospholipids from liver to peripheral tissues.
LDL (Low-density lipoprotein)	Transports cholesterol and phospholipids from liver to tissues and organs like heart.
HDL (High-density lipoprotein)	Transports cholesterol and phospholipids from tissues and organs like heart back to liver.

Low Densityt Lipoprotein (LDL) As"Bad Cholesterol"

Low-density lipoprotein (LDL) is considered as the 'bad cholesterol' because it carries cholesterol and Phospholipids from the liver to different areas of the body Viz. muscles, other tissues and organs such as heart. It is responsible for deposition of cholesterol on walls of arteries causing atherosclerosis (blockage and hardening of the arteries). High levels of LDL (Low-density lipoprotein) increase the risk of heart diseases.

LDL (Low-density lipoprotein) cholesterol typically makes upto 60-70 % of the total serum cholesterol. It contains a single apoliprotein, namely apo B-100 (apo B). LDL (Low-density lipoprotein) is the major atherogenic lipoprotein that has long been identified by NCEP (National cholesterol eradication programme) and considered as the primary target of cholesterol – lowering therapy.

Synthesis of the LDL (Low-density lipoprotein) receptor is regulated by SREBP (Sterol Regulatory Element Binding Protein); the same regulatory protein was used to control the synthesis of cholesterol de novo in response to the cholesterol which is present in the cell. When the cell has abundant cholesterol, LDL (Low-density lipoprotein) receptor synthesis is blocked so that new cholesterol which is formed in the form of LDL (Low-density lipoprotein) molecules cannot be taken up by the cells. On the converse, more LDL (Low-density lipoprotein) receptors are made when the cell is deficient in cholesterol.

When this system is deregulated, many LDL (Low-density lipoprotein) molecules appear in the blood without any receptors on the peripheral tissues. These LDL (Low-density lipoprotein) molecules are oxidized and taken up by the macrophages, which gets engorged and form foam cells. These foam cells often becomes trapped in the walls of blood vessels and contribute to form atherosclerotic plaque formation in the blood vessels. These plaques are the main causes of heart attacks, strokes, and other cardiovascular diseases which lead to the association of so called LDL (Low-density lipoprotein) cholesterol (actually a lipoprotein) with "bad" cholesterol.

High- Density Lipoprotein (HDL) As"Good Cholesterol"

High- density lipoprotein (HDL) is referred as the 'good cholesterol' because it carries cholesterol and phospholipids from tissues and organs back to the liver for degradation and elimination. It prevents the deposition of cholesterol on the walls of arteries, by carrying cholesterol away from arteries to the liver.

High level of HDL (High- density lipoprotein) is a good indicator of a healthy heart, because it reduces the blood cholesterol level. HDL also helps in the normal functioning of some hormones and certain tissues of the body. It is also used for the formation of bile in liver.

HDL (High- density lipoprotein) cholesterol normally makes upto 20-30% of the total serum cholesterol. The major apolipoproteins of HDL (High- density lipoprotein) are apo A-I and apo A-II. HDL –cholesterol levels are inversely correlated with the risk for CHD (Cardiac Heart diseases). HDL (High- density lipoprotein) protects against the development of atherosclerosis, although a low HDL (High- density lipoprotein) level often reflects the presence of other atherogenic factors.

HDL (High- density lipoprotein) particles are thought to transport cholesterol back to the liver for excretion or to other tissues that use cholesterol to synthesize hormones in a process known as reverse cholesterol transport (RCT). Large numbers of large HDL particles can be correlated with better health outcomes. In contrast, having small numbers of large HDL (High- density lipoprotein) particles is independently associated with the atheromatous disease progression within the arteries.

Apolipoproteins:

Apolipoproteins are proteins that bind to fats i.e. - lipids. It is a protein component of lipoprotein that regulates their metabolism. Each of four major groups consists of a family of two or more immunologically distinct proteins. All apolipoproteins are synthesized in the liver but the small quantities are produced in almost all the organs. Apart from stabilizing the lipid part, the protein components have specific functions they are as follows:

Functions:

- Act as a structural components of lipoproteins.
- Recognize the cell membrane surface receptors.
- Activate enzymes involved in lipoprotein metabolism.

Classes:

There are six major classes of apolipoproteins they are:

- A (apo A-I , apo A-II, apo AIV and apo A-V)
- B (apo B48 and apo B100)
- C
- D
- E
- H

Synthesis and regulation:

Apolipoprotein synthesis in the intestine is regulated principally by the fat content of the diet. Apolipoprotein synthesis in the liver is controlled by a host of factors, including dietary composition, hormones i.e. - insulin, glucagon, thyroxin, oestrogens, androgens, alcohol intake and various drugs e.g. statins, niacin and fibric acids. Apo B is an integral Apoprotein whereas the others are peripheral Apoproteins.

2.6 Lipid Transport:

Lipid transport in the human body occurs via two pathways viz;

a) Exogenous pathway.

b) Endogenous pathway.

a) Exogenous pathway (i.e. transport of dietary lipids): It permits the efficient transport of the dietary lipids. Dietary triglycerides are hydrolysed by pancreatic lipases within the intestinal lumen and are emulsified with bile acids to form water soluble micelles. Long chain fatty acids are incorporated into triglycerides and packed with apo-B48, cholesterol esters, retinyl esters, phospholipids and cholesterol to form chylomicrons. Nascent chylomicrons are secreted into the intestinal lymph and delivered directly into the systemic circulation. These particles then encounter lipoprotein lipase (LPL) present in the capillary endothelial surfaces of the adipose tissue, heart and skeletal muscle which hydrolyses them to release free fatty acids. The chylomicron particle progressively shrinks in size as the hydrophobic core is hydrolysed and the hydrophilic lipids on particle surface are transferred to HDL(High- density lipoprotein). This results in the formation of smaller cholesterol ester rich particles known chylomicron remnants.

b) Endogenous pathway (i.e. transport of synthesized lipids): It refers to the hepatic secretion and metabolism of VLDL (Verylow - density lipoprotein) to IDL (Intermediate - density lipoprotein) and LDL(Low - density lipoprotein). VLDL (Verylow - density lipoprotein) particles are synthesized in the liver by packaging of hepatic triglycerides with apoB100, cholesterol esters, phospholipids and vitamin E by the action of MTP (microsomal transfer protein). After secretion into plasma VLDL (Verylow - density lipoprotein) acquires multiple copies of apo E and apo CII. The triglycerides of VLDL (Verylow- density lipoprotein) are hydrolysed by LPL (lipoprotein lipase) in muscle and adipose tissue after which they shrink to become IDL (Intermediate - density lipoprotein) . About 4 to 60% of the VLDL (Verylow - density lipoprotein) remnants and IDLs (Intermediate - density lipoprotein) are removed by the liver by LDL (Low - density lipoprotein) receptor mediated endocytosis via binding to apo E. The remaining IDL (Intermediate - density lipoprotein) is remodelled to form LDL (Low - density lipoprotein) which contains only apo B100. Approximately 70% of LDLs are cleared by LDL (Low - density lipoprotein) mediated receptor endocytosis in the liver.

2.7 Lipids In Diet:

Lipids are mostly consumed in the form of neutral fats, which are also known as triglycerides. Triglycerides are made up of glycerol nucleus and free fatty acids. Triglycerides form the major constituent in foods of animal origin and much less in foods of plant origin. Apart from triglycerides, usual diet also contains small quantities of cholesterol and cholesterol esters.

Dietary fats are classified into two types:

1. Saturated fats.
2. Unsaturated fats.

1. **Saturated fats:** Saturated fats are the fats which contain triglycerides formed from only saturated fatty acids. The fatty acids having maximum amount of hydrogen ions without any double bonds between carbon atoms are called saturated fatty acids.
2. **Unsaturated fats:** Fats containing unsaturated fatty acids are known as unsaturated fats. Unsaturated fatty acids are fatty acids formed by dehydrogenation of saturated fatty acids.

Unsaturated fats are classified into three types:

1. Monosaturated fats
2. Polysaturated fats
3. Trans fats.

1. Monosaturated fats – Unsaturated fats which contain one double bond between the carbon atoms are called monosaturated fats.
2. Polysaturated fats – Unsaturated fats with more than one double bond between the carbon atoms are called polysaturated fats. Polysaturated fats belong to the family of essential fatty acids (fatty acids required in diet).

Polysaturated fats are of two types:

a) Omega -3 fats or omega -3 fatty acids having double bond in the third space from the end of the carbon chain.

b) Omega -6 fats or omega -6 fatty acids having double bond in the sixth space from the end of the carbon chain.

3. Trans fats – Trans fats or fatty acids are unsaturated fatty acids, with molecules containing trans (across or opposite side) double bonds between carbon atoms.

2.8 Digestion Of Lipids:

Lipids are digested by lipolytic enzymes.

Table no-3 Digestion of lipids by various enzymes.

Area	Juice	Enzyme	Substrate	End product
Mouth	Saliva	Lingual lipase	Triglycerides	Fatty acid 1,2 Diacylglycerol
Stomach	Gastric juice	Gastric lipase (weak lipase)	Triglycerides	Fatty acids Glycerol
Small intestine	Pancreatic juice	Pancreatic lipase	Triglycerides	Monoglycerides Fatty acids
		Cholesterol ester hydrolase	Cholesterol ester	Free Cholesterol Fatty acids
		Phospholipase A	Phospholipids	Lysophospholipids
		Phospholipase B	Lysophospholipids	Phosphoryl choline Free fatty acids
		Colipase	Facilitates action of pancreatic lipase	-
	Succus entericus	Bile – salt – activated lipase	Phospholipids Cholesterol esters	Lysophospholipids Cholesterol and fatty acids.
		Intestinal lipase	Triglycerides	Fatty acids Glycerol (weak action)

2.9 Absorption Of Lipids:

Monoglycerides, cholesterol and fatty acids from the micelles enter the cells of intestinal mucosa by simple diffusion.

From here, further transport occurs as follows:

1. In the mucosal cells, most of the monoglycerides are converted into triglycerides. Triglycerides are also formed by re- esterification of fatty acids with more than 10 to12 carbon atoms. Some of the cholesterol is also esterified.
   Triglycerides and cholesterol esters are coated with a layer of protein, cholesterol and phospholipids to form the particles called chylomicrons.

   Chylomicrons cannot pass through the membrane of the blood capillaries because of the larger size. So, these lipid particles enter the lymph vessels and then are transferred into blood from lymph.

2. Fatty acids containing less than 10-12 carbon atoms enter the portal blood from mucosal cells and are transported as free fatty acids or unesterified fatty acids. Most of the fats are absorbed in the upper part of small intestine. Presence of bile is essential for fat absorption.

2.10 Storage Of Lipids:

Lipids are stored in two major tissues:

1. Adipose tissue
2. Liver.

1. Adipose tissue - Fat stored in adipose tissue is called neutral fat or tissue fat. When chylomicrons are traveling through capillaries of adipose tissue or liver, the enzyme called lipoprotein lipase present in the capillary endothelium hydrolyses triglycerides of chylomicrons into free fatty acids (FFA) and glycerol. FFA (free fatty acids) and glycerol enter the fat cells (adipocytes or lipocytes) of the adipose tissue or liver cells. Then, the FFA (free fatty acids) and glycerol are again converted into triglycerides and stored in these cells. When other tissue of the body need energy, triglycerides stored in adipose tissue is hydrolysed into FFA (free fatty acids) and glycerol. FFA (free fatty acids) is transported to the body tissues through blood.

2. Liver – Large quantities of triglycerides appear in the liver during starvation, in diabetes mellitus and in any other condition. Most of the triglycerides are mobilized from the adipose tissue as FFA (free fatty acids) in the blood and then redeposited as a Triglyceride in liver.

Transport Of Lipids In Blood:

Free fatty acids are transported in the blood in combination with albumin. Other lipids are transported in the blood, in the form of lipoproteins.

Table No: 4 Normal Values Of Lipid Profile

Lipids	Desireable Optimaal level	Borderline range	High- risk level
Total Choleterol	<200 mg/dl	200-240mg/dl	>240mg/dl
Triglycerides	<150mg/dl	150-200mg/dl	>200mg/dl
HDL (High density lipoprotein)	>60mg/dl	40-60mg/dl	<40mg/dl
LDL(Lo density lipoprotein)	<60mg/dl	60-100mg/dl	>100mg/dl
Total Cholesterol- HDL ratio	<2	2 to 6	>6

CHAPTER -3 AYURVEDIC REVIEW OF LIPIDS :

3.1- Introduction to Medo Dhatu(Fatty Tissue):

" स्नेहसारोऽयं पुरुष: प्राणाश्च स्नेहभूयिष्ठा: स्नेहसाध्याश्च भवन्ति॥
(सु. चि -३१/१)

The human body is formed from Snehasara (Essence of oiliness). Here Snehasara (Essence of oiliness) means the most Shudhatara(Pure) form of Sneha (Oiliness). The Prana(Life) of human being also depends on Sneha (Oiliness).

Sneha (oiliness) is an attribute that is present in all the Dhatus (Tissues) of the body except Asthi Dhatu (Bone tissue). It is a parameter for the Dhatusaratva (Quality of excellence of all tissues) of all the Dhatus (Tissues) except Asthi Dhatu(Bone tissue). Snehana (Oiling) is mainly the function of Medo Dhatu (fatty tissue) and the same property can also be seen in Vasa (fatty deposits), Majja (bone marrow). These three only differs in their site and function.

Thus, Meda (Fat), Majja(bone marrow) and Vasa (fatty deposits) being predominat in Snigdha (Unctuous), Guru(Heavy) Guna(Property) are qualitatively similar in properties. As Meda (Fat), Majja(bone marrow) and Vasa(fatty deposits) are the major sites where the Sneha (Oiliness) is apparent, the main focus is kept on Medo Dhatu (fatty tissue) as it is significant in lipid metabolism and the resultant pathology.

Lipids can be co related with Medo Dhatu(fatty tissue), Vasa(fatty deposits) and Majja (bone marrow) Dhatu(Tissue). Although they have Snehatwa(oiliness) as a common feature but these three differ in their site and function. Meda(Fat) is present mainly in Udara(Abdomen), but if it is present inside Anu Asthi (Small bone) it is called Sarakta Medas (Fat associated with blood) and when it is in Sthula Asthi (Large bone), the same is called Majja (Bone marrow). The pure form of Medas(fats) present in Mamsa Peshi(Muscle) is called Vasa (Fatty deposits). Thus all the forms of lipids in the body are present mainly in Meda(Fat), Vasa (Fatty deposits), and Majja (Bone marrow). But importance is given to Meda Dhatu(Fatty tissue) as it plays an important role in developing many metabolic disorders like Medoroga(Diseases of Fat), Prameha(Diabetes), etc.

3.2 Etymology And Definition:

Medo Dhatu(Fatty Tissue):

The words Medas and Meda origins from the Sanskrit root word 'Mid' with the addition of 'Asun' and 'Ach' Pratyaya respectively which indicates the meaning of Meda Dhatu(Fatty tissue). Meda(Fat) is also defined as the one which performs the function of Snehana(Oiling). It is a specific type of Dhatu(Tissue) that is originated from the Mamsa Dhatu(Muscle tissue). Vapa and Vasa are the term used synonymously with Medo Dhatu(Fatty tissue).

Vapavahana:

Vapavahana is a site in the abdominal cavity where accumulation of Meda Dhatu(Fatty tissue) occurs.

Vasa (Fatty deposits):

"शुध्दमांसस्य य: स्नेह: सा वसा परिकीर्तिता ।"

(सु. शा. ४/१३)

Vasa (Fatty deposits) is the fat content of the Mamsa Dhatu(Muscle tissue) and is qualitatively similar Medo Dhatu(Fatty tissue). It is the Upadhatu (Subtissue)of Mamsa Dhatu (Muscle tissue)and differs from Meda(Fat) depending upon the site and mode of production.

Majja dhatu (Bone marrow tissue):

Majja(Bone marrow) is the 6th among the seven Dhatus(Tissues) and gets nourishment from Asthi Dhatu (Muscle tissue). It is situated in the hollow surface of bones.

Karma(Functions) of Majja Dhatu(Bone marrow tissue) includes - Imparting Sneha(Oiling) and Bala(Strength) to the body, filling hollow spaces of Asthi(Bone) and nourishment of Shukra Dhatu (Reproductive tissue).

3.3 Sthana(Site) And Swarupa(Form) Of Meda Dhatu(Fatty Tissue):

Meda(Fat) is considered as Sneha(Oil) dominant Drava Dhatu (Liquid tissue) which is having Guru (heavy), Snigdha (oiliness) properties and dominance of Prithvi(Earth), Apa(Water) and Teja(Fire) Mahabhuta(Element).

Meda(Fat) is a yellowish, greasy, soft, solid material; innumerable globules of fat form a thick, spongy layer under the skin.

Site Of Medo Dhatu(Fatty Tissue):

Chakrapani has classified all the Dhatus(Tissues) into two types. On the basis of function of Poshana (Nourishment), Medo Dhatu(Fatty tissue)can be categorized into two types:

1. Poshya Medo Dhatu (Nourished Fatty tissue)/ Baddha Meda(Formed Fat)
2. Poshaka Medo Dhatu(Nutrient Fatty tissue) / Abaddha Meda(Unformed Fat)

1. **Poshya Medo Dhatu**(Nourished Fatty tissue) / **Baddha Meda**(Formed Fat) - The Sthayi(Stable) or Poshya Medo Dhatu (Nourished Fatty tissue) is derived from the Poshaka Medo Dhatu (Nutrient Fatty tissue) by the action of Medodhatvagni(Fatty tissue metabolic fire). It is immobile in nature (Gativivarjita) and is stored in Medodharakala which is situated in Udara(Abdomen) and Anuasthi(Small bone). Udara(Abdomen), Sphika(Gluteal), Stana(Breast), Gala(Neck) are also depots of Poshya Meda(Nourished fat) as seen in Atisthaulya(Excessive obesity).

2. **Poshaka Medo Dhatu**(Nutrient Fatty tissue) / **Abaddha Meda**(Unformed Fat) - The Poshaka Medo Dhatu being Asthayi(Unstable) in nature circulates along with the Rasa(Plasma) Rakta(Blood) to give nutition to the Sthayi Poshya Medo Dhatu(Stable Nourished Fatty tissue). It is mobile in nature (Gatiyukta).

3.4 Composition And Attributes Of Medo Dhatu(Fatty tissue):

Composition of Medo Dhatu:

" मेदो जलपृथिव्यात्मकम् ।"

(सु. सु. १५/८ चक्रपाणि)

Though Medo Dhatu(Fatty tissue) is Panchabhautika(Penta elemental) in nature, it is mainly composed of Pruthvi(Earth) and Apa(Water) Mahabhutas(Elements).

Attributes of medo dhatu:

Meda Dhatu is Atisnigdha(Excessive unctuous), Guru(Heavy), Sthula(Bulkiness), Pichchila(Sticky), Mridu(Soft), Sandra(Solidity). It is also white in colour.

3.5 Karma(Functions) Of Meda Dhatu (Fatty Tissue):

" मेद: स्नेहस्वेदौ दृढत्वं पुष्टिमस्थ्नां च ।"

(सु.सु -१५/७)

"नेत्रगात्रस्निग्धतास्नेहदाढर्यास्थिपुष्टिभिर्मेद: ।"

(अ.सं.सु -१९/४)

The main functions of Meda Dhatu(Fatty tissue) are as follows:

1. **Snehana (oiliness)** – Sneha(Oiling) quality helps to maintain the luster of skin, hairs, eyes and various body organs. Snigdhagatrata(Unctous Body) arise in Medoroga(Diseases of Fat) may be due to increased Snehana(Oiliness) function of Meda(Fat).

2. **Sweda (sweat)** – It is also known a mala(Waste) of Meda Dhatu(Fatty tissue). The function of Meda(Fat) is to produce Sweda(Sweat). According to Acharya Sharangdhara, Sweda(Sweat) is the Upadhatu(Subtissue) of Meda Dhatu(Fatty tissue).

3. **Drudhatva (strength)** - Meda Dhatu(Fatty tissue) provides Dhrudhata to the body. Snayu(Tendon) is the Upadhatu(Subtissue) of Meda(Fat). Snayu(Tendon) provides support to Asthi(Bone) and Sandhi(Joints) and helps in joint formation. Meda(Fat) also provides support to various organs and helps in binding of organs. The fat tissue deposits as a layer over underlying organ thereby providing it protection from outside pressure and frictions.

4. **Asthi Pushti (strengthening of bones)** - Meda Dhatu(Fatty tissue) another function is to nourish the subsequent Dhatu(Tissue) i.e. Asthi (Bone) and its Upadhatu(Subtissue) Snayu(Tendons) and Sandhi(Joints). It also lubricates the Asthi(Tendon) and Sandhi(Joints) thus minimizing their friction.

5. **Netra and Gatra Snigdhata (oiliness of eyes and body)** - Both are the symptoms of Sthaulya(Obesity) and may arise through increased Snehana(oiliness) function of Meda(Fat).

3.6 Medovaha Srotas (Channels Of Fatty Tissue):

" स्रोतांसि खलु परिणाममापद्यमानानां धातूनामभिवाहीनि भवन्त्ययनार्थेन ।"

(च. वि.- ५/३)

As observed by Acharya Charaka, "Nutrients substances which nourish the Dhatu(Tissue) undergo Paka(Transformation) by the Ushma(Hotness) of Dhatus (Dhatwagni) (Tissue fire). Then they are made available to the Dhatus(Tissues) through their own Srotas (Channels)." The Srotas(Channels) which provide nutrition to the Meda Dhatu(Fatty tissue) or the Srotas(Channels) carrying the nutritive contents to the site of Meda Dhatu(Fatty tissue) can be considered as Medovaha Srotas (Channels of Fatty tissue).

According to C. Dwarkanath, the channels through which nutrition to the adipose tissue is transported are to be termed as Medovaha Srotas(Channels of Fatty tissue). Vitiation of Medovaha Srotas(Channels of Fatty tissue) takes place in Medodushti(Vitiation of Fat) or Medoroga (Diseases of Fat).

Formation Of Meda Dhatu From Raktadi Dhatus:

Meda Dhatu(Fatty tissue) forms from Mamsa Dhatu(Muscle tissue) when acted upon by Meda Dhatvagni(Fat etabolic tissue fire) on Medaposhakansha (Nutrients of fat). Any disturbance found in above pathways during formation of Meda Dhatu (Fatty tissue) , may lead to Medo Dushti(Vitiation of fat) i.e. either Vruddhi or Kshaya(Increase or decrease) of Meda Dhatu(Fatty tissue).

3.7 Derangement Of Meda(Fat) Metabolism:

Agni(Metabolic Fire) is responsible for all the metabolic activities of the body. It is solely responsible for any increase or decrease of Dosha(Bodily humor), Dhatu(Tissue) or Mala(Waste).The vitiation of Agni(Metabolic Fire) has serious impact on health at various levels depending on type of Agni(Metabolic Fire) involved.

When Agni(Metabolic Fire) is decreased, it will lead to various metabolic disorders at various levels and produces "Ama" (undigested materials) i.e. Agni(Metabolic Fire) fails to convert the Vijatiya (non-assimilable) Dravyas(Substance) into Sajatiya (assimilable) ones and the end products cannot be assimilated by the Dhatus(Tissue).

If Agnimandya (Impairement in Metabolic Fire) is present at the level of Jatharagni(Digestive fire) only, then Ama(Undigested food) is usually restricted to koshtha (Abdomen). There will be no production of Ahara Rasa(Essence of food) and result will be Dhatu Kshaya (Decrease in tissue).

If Agnimandya(Impairement in Metabolic Fire) is present at the level of Bhutagni(Elemental fire), then Ama(Undigested food) is restricted to Ahara Rasa(Essence of food) and this Ahara rasa(Essence of food) which is improperly formed cannot be assimilated by Dhatus(Tissues) and results in Dhatukshaya(Decrease in tissue). The Ama (Undigested food) which is in circulation can be accumulated in any parts of the body leading to various disorders. Out of 5 Bhutagni (Elemental fire) which one is involved is also important to note. If one Bhutagni(Elemental fire) is involved, it leads to impairement in nourishment of that particular Dhatu(Tissue) which is having predominance of that particular Mahabhuta(Element).

If Agnimandya(Impairement in Metabolic Fire) is present at the level of Dhatvagni(Tissue metabolic fire) (one or more), then the particular Dhatus(Tissues) cannot assimilate nutrients present in the circulating Ahara rasa(Essence of food) or cirulating Poshaka Dhatu (Nutrient tissue). So, such Poshaka Dhatus(Nutrient tissue) will be accumulated in Ahara rasa(Essence of food) in abnormal quantities and further they may get accumulated at abnormal sites. This sort of process can be called leenatwa (deep seated) of Ama(Undigested food) in Dhatus(Tissues).

Once Jatharagni(Digestive fire) is impaired, the Bhutagni(Elemental fire) and Dhatvagni(Tissue metabolic fire) would also get impaired. Hence during treatment of any kind of

Agnimandya(impairement in Metabolic fire) or Ama (Undigested food)conditions, one should think about all the three levels.

When Medo Dhatvagni (Fatty tissue fire) is impaired and the homologues nutrients present in Poshaka Medo Dhatu(Nutirent fat tissue) will be in excess in circulation and this can be referred to the conditions such as hyperlipidaemia. This is because the Poshaka Medo Dhatu(Nutirent fat tissue) cannot be assimilated into Sthayi Medo Dhatu(Stable fat tissue) by Medo Dhatwagni(Fatty tissue fire). The cause for excess Poshaka Medo Dhatu(Fatty tissue fire) in circulation is not only the Medo Dhatwagnimandya(impairement in fatty tissue fire), but there may be decrease in other Agni(Metabolic Fire) also. Any cause, which can lead to Kapha Vriddhi (Increase in phlegm), Pitta Kshaya(Decrease in fire) or Vata Prakopa(Aggravation in air), can lead to this condition.

The consequence of such increase in Poshaka Medo Dhatu(Nutirent fat tissue) may be Dhamani Pratichaya(Atherosclerosis). The excess Poshaka Medo Dhatu (Nutirent fat tissue) may accumulate on the walls of vessels (Dhamani) and may cause serious complications related to circulation. Dhamani Pratichaya(Atherosclerosis) is considered as one of the Nanatmaja Kapha Roga(Diseases of Phlegm).

3.8 Pathophysiology Of Meda Dhatu(Fatty Tissue):

The formation of a Dhatu(Tissue) from the four types of ingested Ahara(Food) takes place after the digestion by Jatharagni(Digestive fire). Jatharagni(Digestive fire) is the main metabolic principle that is mainly responsible for giving strength to the Bhutagnis(Elemental fire) as well as the Dhatvagnis(Tissue fire). Optimal functioning of Dhatvagni(Tissue fire) leads to the qualitatively as well as quantitatively properly formed Meda Dhatu(Fatty tissue). The Vyan Vayu(Air) is the force of transportation which provides the nutrient material to the various tissues. Also those Srotas(Channels) through which Dhatus(Tissues) undergoes transformation are required to be in an unimpaired state, as any impairement in the Srotas(Channels) will lead to an impaired Dhatu(Tissue) and viceversa.

Agni(Metabolic fire):

Agni(Metabolic Fire) is the one which is responsible for all the metabolic activities occurring in the body. It is the solely responsible for any increase or decrease of the Dhatus(Tissues). Any ingested substances either derived from plants or animals are Vijatiya in nature or dissimilar to the body. Therefore it is essential to transform them into Sajatiya substances or the substances that are similar to the body constituents for their easily assimilation in the body. For this the substances have to undergo metabolism at three different levels of Agni(Metabolic Fire) i.e. – Jatharagni(Digestive fire), Bhutagni(Elemental fire), and Dhatvagni(Tissue fire). Impairement at any of these three levels of Agni(Metabolic Fire) will leads to an impairement in Dhatu(Tissue) formation which results in the formation in either qualitative or quantitatively inferior Dhatu(Tissue) formation.

Jatharagnipaka(Gastrointestinal digestion):

Jatharagnipaka(Gastrointestinal digestion) is meant the digestion of food under the influence of Jatharagni(Digestive fire). Jatharagnipaka (Gastrointestinal digestion) describes the intestinal digestion and the processes involved in it. All types of ingested food undergo Jatharagnipaka (Gastrointestinal digestion) at the outset. The term Jatharagni(Digestive fire) is used synonymously with the Pachaka pitta. The action of Jatharagni (Digestive fire). occurs at a gross level in the Grahani (Duodenum).

The main characteristic of Jatharagni(Digestive fire) is to do Sanghatabheda or disintegration of large particles of food to make it ready for absorption. Thus, Jatharagni(Digestive fire) performs both the function of digestion and absorption of food.

The entire process of digestion has been described the heading of Avasthapaka(Stage of Digestion) which constitutes the Madhurapaka (salivary), Amlapaka (gastric) and Katupaka (intestinal) digestion. Thus the food which is processed further available for the action of Bhutagni (Elemental fire) and Dhatvagni(Tissue fire) .

Jatharagni(Digestive fire) is also the main source of metabolism occurring in the body as any increase or decrease in it leads to an increase or decrease in Bhutagnis(Elemental fire) and Dhatvagnis(Tissue fire). A properly digested substrate formed by the Jatharagni(Digestive fire) is the prerequisite for digestion by Bhutagnis(Elemental fire) and Dhatvagnis(Tissue fire) .

Contemplating upon the lipid metabolism, Jatharagnipaka(Gastrointestinal Digestion) can be referred to as the action lingual lipase and gastric lipase present in the saliva and stomach respectively. Both these enzymes split the fats into fatty acids and glycerol which can be considered as Sanghatabheda (Disintegration) of the ingested lipids. These acts only on fats that are already split up into colloidal droplets. Amashaya (Stomach) moves to the Grahani(Duodenum) where it undergoes emulsification by bile salts to prepare it for the action of water soluble enzymes. Then the emulsified fat is split into fatty acids and glycerol under the influence of pancreatic and intestinal lipase. These fatty acids and glycerol are again taken up by the epithelial cells of the intestine to form new triglycerides that are released as chylomicrons in the lymph.

Jatharagnipaka(Gastrointestinal Digestion) activates Bhutagnis(Element fire) by supplying them with a properly formed substrate which constitutes the second level of digestion.

<u>Bhutagnipaka(Elemental fire digestion):</u>

Bhutagnipaka (Elemental fire digestion) follows Jatharagnipaka(Gastrointestinal Digestion) and it completes the process of intestinal digestion. It is only after the completion of Bhutagnipaka(Elemental fire digestion) that formation of Ahara rasa(essence food) is completed and Rasa Shoshan(Absorption of plasma) is possible. After the action of Jatharagni(Digestive fire) action of Bhutagni(Elemental fire) occurs on the substrate that completes process of intestinal digestion of lipids. The function of bhutagni(Elemental fire) is to make already digested food more assimilable and to ready for the action of Dhatvagnis(Tissue fire). The lipids being Apa Mahabhuta

(Water element) and Prithvi Mahabhuta(Earth element) dominant are acted upon by Apyagni(Water fire) and Parthivagni(Earth fire) in the intestine.

The bhutagnipaka(Elemental fire digestion) occurs in liver. The action of liver is to breakdown fats derived from both plants and animal sources to their elemental form and rebuild them in the body in the form of lipids. Cholesterol is primarily synthesized within the body (endogenous) production in the liver from acetyl CoA through the HMG- CoA reductase pathway. Similarly the liver also synthesizes phospholipids, triglycerides and other categories of lipids. This synthesis of different categories of body lipids by liver which are easily assimilable within the body cells may be known as the action of the bhutagnis(Element fire).

Dhatvagnipaka(Tissue fire digestion):

"आमाशयगत: पाकमाहार: प्राप्य केवलम् ।

पक्व: सर्वाश्रयं पश्चाद्धमनीभि: प्रपद्यते॥" (च.वि.-२/१८)

According to Acharya Charak, the Sarabhaga(Essence part) or the Annarasa(food juice) of the ingested food which is the outcome of the action of both the Jatharagni(Tissue fire) and bhutagnipaka(Elemental fire digestion) is absorbed from Adhoamashya(Pyloric stomach) and is distributed throughout the body by Dhamanis(Vessels).

Role of vata(air):

"कृत्स्नदेहचरो व्यानो रससंवहनोद्यत: ।
स्वेदासृक्स्त्रावणश्चापि पञ्चधा चेष्टयत्यपि ॥
क्रुद्धश्च कुरूते रोगान् प्रायश: सर्वदेहगान् ।"
(सु.नि.-१/१७-१८)

Here Maruta(Air) refers to mainly to the vyana vayu, as it is the main transport vehicle for the circulation of Ahara rasa(Essence food) in the body. Although the main seat of Vyana Vayu(Air) is Hridaya(Heart), its main site of action is entire body. The vitiation of Vyana Vayu(Air) results in diseases pertaining to the entire body. Vyana Vayu (Air) is the driving force which is responsible for the circulation of lipoproteins throughout the body.

Role of Srotas(Channels):

"कुपितानां हि दोषाणां शरीरे परिधावताम् ।
यत्र सङ्गः खवैगुण्याव्द्याधिस्तत्रोपजायते ॥"
(सु.नि.-२४/१९)

The Srotas are the channels in the body in which the transportation of Asthayi Dhatu(Unstable tissue) takes place which leads to the formation of Sthayi Dhatu(Stable tissue). Acharya Sushruta has explained the major role of Srotas(Channels) in pathogenesis. Similarly the main defect in the Medovaha Srotas(Channels of Fatty tissue) is responsible for the pathogenesis taking place in hyperlipidaemia.

3.9 Pathological Conditions Meda Dhatu (Fatty tissue) :

Medo pradoshaja vikara (Diseases of Fat)–

"मेद: संश्रयास्तुं प्रचक्ष्मेह । निन्दितानि प्रमेहाणां पूर्वरुपाणि यानि च ।"

(च. सु. -२८/१५)

The prodromal symptoms of Prameha(Diabetes) Jatilibhava Keseshu(tortuous hair), much Madhurya(more sweetness), Kara-Pada Suptata and Daha(Numbness and Burning in hands – feet), etc and the Ashto Nindita(Eight undesirable) Personalities i.e- Ati Deergha(Excessive tall), Ati Hrasva(Excessive short), Ati Loma(Excessive body hairs), Aloma(Absence of hairs), Atikrishna(Excessive black), Ati gaur(Excessive white), Ati Sthula(Excessive obese), Ati Krusha(Excessive lean) are caused due to the vitiation of Medo Dhatu(Fatty tissue) and Medovaha Srotas(Channels of fatty tissue).

Meda Vriddhi (Increase of fat) –

"मेद:स्निग्धाङ्गतामुदरपार्श्ववृद्धिं कासश्वासादीन् दौर्गन्ध्यं च ।"(सु. सु. -१५/१९)

Excessive formation of Meda Dhatu(Fatty tissue) leads to oiliness and stickiness in body parts, increased abdominal girth, Cough, dyspnea on exertion and foul body odour.

Sthaulya (Obesity)-

Accumulation of Medo(Fat) leading to enlargement of the abdomen (adiposity).

Medodosha(Excessive fatness) –

Excessive Meda(Fat) leading to the obstruction of Srotamsi (Lipid disorder leading to atherosclerosis and its complication). Kshudra Shwaas or dyspnea on exertion and Moha or syncope, the cardinal symptoms of coronary and cerebral insufficiency are the examples of Medo Dosha(Excessive fatness).

CHAPTER- 4 MODERN DISEASE REVIEW OF HYPERLIPIDAEMIA:

4.1- Introduction Of Hyperlipidaemia:

Lipid and lipoprotein abnormalities are extremely commom in the general population and are regarded as a highly modifiable risk factor for cardiovascular disease due to the influence of cholesterol, one of the most clinically relevant lipid substances on atherosclerosis. Hyperlipidaemia is the term used to denote raised serum levels of one or more of the total cholesterol, triglycerides, low density lipoprotein, high density lipoprotein or combination of both. The abnormal levels of Triglycerides and /or cholesterol in plasma are consequent to excess of substrate leads to more production, defective transport, delayed peripheral clearance, reduced utilization of lipoproteins or their intermediaries, or combinations of these abnormalities.

Dyslipidaemia is an abnormal amount of lipids in the blood. In developed countries, most dyslipidemias are hyperlipidaemias; that is, an elevation of lipids in the blood, often due to diet and lifestyle. The prolonged elevation of insulin levels can lead to dyslipidaemia. Hyperlipidaemia or hyperlipoproteinemia is the condition of abnormally elevated levels of any or all lipids and or lipoproteins in the blood.

4.2 Classification:

Hyperlipidaemia is classified in two distinct ways:

1. Phenotypically – Fredrickson and levy classified Hyperlipoproteinaemias according to the type of lipoprotein particles that accumulate in the blood.
2. Etiologically – Depending on underlying cause, i.e. a) Primary (genetic) or b) Secondary (due to another condition).

Table No 5 : Fredrickson Classification (Phenotypic) of Hyperlipidaemia:

Phenotype	Lipoprotein elevated	Lipid elevated	Atherogenecity
I (Familial lipoprotein lipase deficiency	Chylomicrons	Tg ↑↑↑ Chol N to ↑	Not known
II-a (Familial hypercholesterolaemia)	LDL	Tg N Chol ↑↑	Very high
II-b Polygenic Hypercholesterolaemia	VLDL and LDL	Tg ↑↑ Chol ↑↑	Very high
III Familial dysbeta-Lipoproteinaemia	IDL (Remnants)	Tg ↑↑↑ Chol ↑↑	Very high
IV Hypertriglycerid - eamia	VLDL	Tg ↑↑ Chol N to ↑	High
V Familial combined Hyperlipidaemia	VLDL and Chylomicrons	Tg ↑↑↑↑ Chol ↑/↑↑	Higher

N	Normal Level	↑↑↑	Severely raise
↑	Mild Raised	↑↑↑↑	Very Severely raised
↑↑	Moderately raised	Tg	Triglycerides
Chol	Cholesterol	VLDL	Very low density lipoprotein
LDL	Low density cholesterol	HDL	High density lipoprotein
IDL	Intermediate density lipoprotein		

BASED ON ETIOLOGY

1. **Primary dyslipidaemia -** It may be expressed in the form of familial syndromes. About 60% variability in the serum fasting lipids may be genetically determined. Genetic defects lead to accumulation in the plasma of excessive amounts of lipoproteins usually due to the failure of catabolic apparatus and seldom due to accumulation of lipoproteins caused by increased synthesis.

Primary Causes of Hyperlipidaemias:

I) Hypercholesterolaemia-

Monogenic

- Familial hypercholesterolaemia due to decreased clearance of LDL (low density lipoprotein).
- Familial combined hyperlipidaemia – excess of Triglycerides and apoprotein B-100 prodution.
- Familial monogenic hypercholesterolaemia due to over production of apoprotein B-100.

Polygenic hypercholesterolaemia.

II) Hypertriglyeridaemia-

Over production of VLDL (Very low density lipoprotein) & Triglycerides -

- Familial endogenous hypertriglyceridaemia without excess apoprotein B -100 prodution.
- Familial combined hyperlipidaemia (as above).

Peripheral clearance defect of Triglyceride-rich Lipoproteins

- Familial LP: deficiency (Fredrickson Type-1)
- Familial apoprotein C –II deficiency

Primary clearance defects

- Familial endogenous hypertriglyceridaemia.
- Familial Type V hyperlipoproteinaemia.
- Familial combined hyperlipidaemia- clearance defect with excess apoprotein B-48 production.

2. **Secondary hyperipidaemia –**

Secondary causes contribute to most cases of Dyslipidaemia in adults. The most important secondary cause in developed countries is a sedentary lifestyle with excessive dietary intake of saturated fat, cholesterol, and Trans fats.

Table No 6 : Causes of Secondary Hyperlipidaemia:

HYPERCHOLESTEROLAEMIA	**HYPERTRIGLYCERIDAEMIA**
Hypothyroidism	Obesity
Diabetes mellitus	Diabetes mellitus
Cushing's Syndrome	Hypothyroidism
Oral contraceptives	Diet rich in carbohydrates
Diet rich in saturated fat	Excessive alcohol consumption
Nephrotic syndrome	Chronic renal failure
Chronic liver disease	Cushing's Syndrome
Anorexia nervosa	Beta- blockers and diuretics
Acute intermittent porphyria	Glucocorticoid and estrogen use
Cholestasis	Dysglobulinaemia
Dysglobulinaemia	Systemic lupus erythematosus
	Hypopituitarism
	Pregnancy

4.3 Signs And Symptoms :

HYPERCHOLESTEROLAEMIA	HYPERTRIGLYCERIDAEMIA
Xanthelasma of eyelid	Lipaemia retinalis
Corneal arcus	Eruptive xanthoma
Xanthomata of palms, knee and elbows	Acute pancreatitis
Atheromatous plaques in arteries	Hepatosplenomegaly
Myocardial infarction	

4.4 Complications :

Hyperlipidaemia since the pathogenesis proceeds further depending on various other factors like the site of localization etc. The main importance of the disease Hyperlipidaemia lies on its ability to cause several complications which are as follows.

1. Premature Coronary Artery Disease
2. Heart Attack
3. Stroke
4. Pancreatitis
5. Atherosclerosis

High lipid levels due to a buildup of plaque can increase the rate at which sticky, fatty sticky, fatty deposits known as plaque buildup in the body. In addition to reducing the blood flow through the arteries, the plaque also causes the arteries to harden, making them less flexible. This condition is known as atherosclerosis and can contribute to heart disease and possibly heart attack.

4.5 Management Of Hyperlipidaemia According To Modern Science:

The general approach to the management of hyperlipidaemia is organized into four components:

- Assessment and monitoring of disease severity and control to reduce cardiovascular risk.
- Patient education and self-management about the disease process, lifestyle modifications, and medication use.
- Mitigation of comorbidities that increase cardiovascular risk such as diabetes, hypertension, smoking, and HAART treatment of HIV disease, as well as management of existing coronary artery disease, stroke, and peripheral vascular diseas.e
- Medications including statins, fibrates, etc.

Treatment Strategy Of Hyperlipidaemia:

Treatment strategy

Non Pharmacological Management → **Preventive Measures**

1. Dietary Suggestions
2. Lifestyle Modifications

Main cornerstone of therapy in Hyperlipidaemia

Pharmacological Management → **Internal Medication**

Non Pharmacological Management:

1. **Dietary Suggestions-** Includes
   - Increase intake of high fibre foods- e.g Oat meal, Vegetables, Salads,etc.
   - Restrict saturated fat intake- e.g. meat, dairy products, cheese, fried foods, butter, etc.
   - Dietary protein with low fat content could be selected- e.g.- dried beans, peas, pulses.
   - Diet should contain- green tea, nuts , onions, garlic, etc.
   - Avoid sugar and refined grain products, packed and processed foods.
   - Avoid intake of excessive alcohol and caffeine.

2. **Lifestyle Modifications-**
   - Weight reduction- is the key strategy specially in obese patients.
   - Cessation of smoking.
   - Physical activity.

Pharmacological Management :

Drug Classifications:

1. **HMG – CoA reductase inhibitors (Statins):**

   Lovastatin, Simvastatin, Pravastatin, Atorvastatin, Rosuvastatin.
2. **Bile acid sequestrants (Resins):**

   Cholestyramine , Colestipol.
3. **Activate lipoprotein lipase (Fibric acid derivatives):**

   Clofibrate, Gemfibrozil, Bezafibrate, Fenofibrate.
4. **Inhibit lipolysis and triglyceride synthesis :**

   Nicotinic acid.
5. **Others:** Ezetimibe, Gugulipid.

Table No 7: Summary Of Major Drugs Used For The Treatment Of Hyperlipidaemia:

Drug	Major Indications	Mechanism	Common side Effects
HMG-CoA reductase inhibitors Lovastatin Pravastatin Simvastatin Fluvastatin Atorvastatin	Elevated LDL (low density lipoprotein)	Decrease cholesterol synthesis, decrease hepatic LDL (low density lipoprotein) receptors, decrease VLDL (Verylow density lipoprotein) production	Myalgias Artralgias Elevated transaminases Dyspepsia
Bile acid sequestrants Cholestyramine Colestipol Colesevelam	Elevated LDL (low density lipoprotein)	Increase bile excretion and increase LDL receptor	Bloating Constipation Elevated Triglycerides
Nicotinic acid Immediate release Sustained release Extended release	Elevated LDL (low density lipoprotein) , HDL (High density lipoprotein) , elevated Triglycerides	Decrease hepatic VLDL(Verylow density lipoprotein) synthesis	Cutaneous flushing GI upset Elevated glucose, uric acid and other liver function test
Fibric acid derivatives Gemfibrizol Fenofibrate	Elevated Triglycerides, elevated remnants	Increase LPL (lipoprotein lipase), decrease hepatic VLDL (Verylow density lipoprotein) synthesis	Dispepsia Myalgia Gallstones Elevated Transaminases
Fish oils	Severely elevated Triglycerides	Decrease chylomicron and VLDL(Verylow density lipoprotein) production	Dyspepsia Diarrhea Fishy odour to Breath
Cholesterol absorption inhibitors Ezetimibe	Elevated LDL (low density lipoprotein)	Decrease intestinal cholesterol absorption	Elevated Transaminase

CHAPTER 5 -AYURVEDIC DISEASE REVIEW OF HYPERLIPIDAEMIA :

5.1 Hyperlipidaemia in Ayurveda:

Hyperlipidaemia does not bear a precise reference in Ayurveda though the study of Ayurvedic literature bears some implicit allusions. This might be due to the fact that it is a metabolic disorder and not a full fledged disease in itself. It is supplementary to several other severe conditions like coronary artery disease, cerebrovascular accidents, metabolic syndrome etc.

In Ayurveda various attempts have been made to use distinctive nomenclature to denote the word hyperlipidaemias which are as follows:

1. Rasagat Sneha Vriddhi (Increase of unctuousness in plasma)
2. Rasa Raktagat Sneha Vriddhi (Increase of unctuousness in plasma & blood)
3. Medovriddhi (Increase in fat)
4. Medoroga or Medodosha (Disease of fat or Excessive fat)
5. Ama Medo Dhatu (unriped / immature fatty tissue)

The study of Ayurvedic literature bears certain uncertain references pertaining to an increase in the amount of circulating body lipids, yet the literal meaning of Hyperlipidaemia is not found to be distinctly stated anywhere. The study of Hyperlipidaemia can be done on the basis of studying three of the closest diseases in the Ayurveda having same amount of relation with hyperlipidaemia are:

1. Atisthaulya (Excessive Obesity)
2. Medo Roga (Fatty disease)
3. Prameha (Diabetes)

According to Ayurvedic view Pitta or Agni (metabolic fire) is responsible for all transformations in the body. If Agni (metabolic fire) of any part is impaired the proper transformation of body constituents in that part is affected. As a result either faulty transformation will take place or transformation is arrested and materials for transformation accumulate in that part. The factors responsible for Agni (metabolic fire) vitiation may be congenital or acquired.

Dhatwagni Vaigunya (weak tissue metabolic fire) is the causative factor of hyperlipidaemia. Due to this Dhatu Parinama (proper conversion of tissue) is affected. Here

Medodhatu (fatty tissue) is not formed properly. Ama (unriped material) is formed and combined with Dhatus (tissues) so that both Poshaka (nutrient) and Poshya (nourished) part of Dhatu (tissue) became Sama mala (waste substances associated with ama).

Level of various lipids in the body may increase or accumulate by three reasons –

1. Due to complete Dhatwagni Vikriti (Vitiation of tissue metabolic fire) Sthayi Meda Dhatu (stable fatty tissue) is not formed so Poshakans(nutrients) accumulate and combine with Ama (unriped substance).
2. Due to partial Agni Vikriti (Vitiation in metabolic fire) the transformation is partial and Ama (unriped substance) is formed so the formed Dhatu (tissue) and Poshakams (nutrients) will not be normal and become Sama (waste substances with ama).
3. When the intake of Kaphakara (Phlegm forming) and Medokara (fat forming) food is increased continuously, then the Poshakamsa (nutrients) is markedly increased. Even though the Agni (metabolic fire) is normal, due to the overloading of Poshakamsa (nutrients) Agni (metabolic fire) will be unable to convert them to proper Poshya Dhatu (nutritious tissue). Due to accumulation of nutrients Ama (unriped/ immature substance) is formed. This overloading and formation of Ama (unriped/ immature substance) cause formation of Sama Medo Dhatu (unriped fatty tissue). This again vitiates the Agni (metabolic fire) and the condition is worsened.

Accumulated materials in hyperlipdaemia are not proper Dhatu (tissue) and produced due to faulty metabolism. So we can call them as Vikritta Meda Dhatu (Abnormal fatty tissue) and the condition is known as Medo Dhatu Dushti (Vitiated fatty tissue).

Hyperlipidaemia occurs due to-

1. Agnimandya (Impaired metabolic fire)
2. Ama utpatti (Formation of unriped substance)
3. Medoroga (Fatty disease)

5.2 Role Of Agnimandya (Impaired Metabolic Fire) In Hyperlipidaemia:

- The vitiation of Agni (metabolic fire) has serious impact on health at various levels depending on type of Agni(metabolic fire) involved.
- All metabolic diseases are an outcome of improper functioning of Agni(metabolic fire).
- The imbalance in the functional capacity of Agni(metabolic fire) is the main initiating factor for the production of Ama (unriped substance).

5.3 Concept Of Ama (Unriped /Undigested Substance):

"उष्मणोऽल्पबलत्वेन धातुमाद्यमपचितम ।

दुष्टमामाशयगतं रसमामं प्रचक्षते ॥"

(अ . ह. सू १३/२५)

- Ama (unriped substance) is a product of incomplete digestion of food which can be absorbed from GI tract but cannot be utilized by the body cells.
- Ama (unriped substance) formation occurs when intake of food exceeds the digestive capacity i.e. – Agni (metabolic fire).
- Ama (unriped substance) circulates all over the body along with rasa i.e. – body fluids.

PHYSICAL PROPERTIES OF AMA(UNRIPED /UNDIGESTED SUBSTANCE) :

"अविपक्कमसयुक्तम दुर्गन्धं बहु पिच्छलम

सदनं सर्वगात्राणामाम इत्याभिधियत II"

(मा. नि. २५/३)

Ama (unriped substance) has following Qualities- i.e.-

- Dravatvam (Fluidity)
- Gurutvam (heaviness)
- Snighdhatvam (Unctuous)
- Nanavarna (Different colour shades)
- Pichchilatvam (Sticky)
- Tantumatvam (Filamentous)
- Asamyuktama (Unformed)
- Durghandhitvam (Bad odour).

5.4 Dhamani Pratichaya (Atherosclerosis) :

- Dhamani Pratichaya(Atherosclerosis) is considered as one of the Nanatmaja Kapha Roga(Diseases of Phlegm).
- According to Acharya Charak it is Kaphaja Nanatmaja Vyadhi (Charak Samhita)
- The excess Poshaka Medo Dhatu may accumulate on the walls of vessels (Dhamani) and may cause serious complications related to circulation.
- In Charak Samhita Sutrasthana chapter 20/17, Acharya Charak has clearly mentioned a term "Dhamanipratichaya" in twenty Kaphaja Nanatmaja Vikaras. On the basis of their clinical manifestations Dhamanipratichaya (Dhamaniupalepa , Dhamanipustata, and Dhamanimatipoorana) can be correlated with the term Atherosclerosis / Arteriosclerosis.

5.5 Nidana Panchak Of Hyperlipidaemia:

Nidana (Etiology):

In hyperlipidaemia the impaired kapha Dosha (Phlegm) and Medo Dhatu (Fatty tissue) are also found to play key role in the pathogenesis of Atisthaulya (Excessive obesity) and Prameha (Diabetes). Hence the causative Nidanas (Etiology) of the later diseases can be also understood as the causative factors of hyperlipidaemia.

Medoroga (hyperlipidaemia) is Santarpanjanya Roga (Overnutrition disease). Nidana (Etiology) of kaphavriddhi (Increase of Phlegm), Medovridhi (increase of fat), Prameha (Diabetes) and Sthaulya (Obesity) are almost similar and they are the Nidana (Etiology) of hyperlipidaemia also. Ahara (Dietetics), Vihara (daily regime) and Beejadushti (Sperm & Ovum defect) are at first sight etiological components. The etiological approach to lipid disorder is a collective attribute derived from the causes (Nidana) of the following conditions i.e – Santarpanjanya Vyadhi(Diseases due to overnutrition), Prameha(Diabeties), Sthaulya(Obesity), and Rasa- Medovaha Srotodushti(Vitiation of channels of plasma and fat).

"मेदो जनयति विशिष्टाहारवशाददृष्टवशान्मेदसाऽऽवृतमार्गत्वाच्च धातुद्वयमतिक्रमय मेद एव वर्धयति ।"

(सु.सु -१५/३२ (डल्हण))

Acharya Dalhana has quoted three main etiological factors of Sthaulya(Obesity) which encompass all the causes leading to an increase in the Asathayi Medo Dhatu (Unstable fatty tissue) thereby leading to a state of hyperlipidaemia.

1. Vishista aharavashat (Specific Dietary factors) :

It refers to the use of specific dietary, lifestyle and psychological factors which lead to Medo Roga (fatty disease). These factors either due to similarity in the attributes or in the action result in a direct increase in Medo Dhatu (fatty tissue) by following Samanya Siddhanta (Principles of similarity).

The causes of Medovaha Srotodushti (Vitiation in fatty tissue channels) can also be considered as etiological factors for hyperlipidaemia, as any derangement in the Srotas (channels) leads to the Dhatu Dushti (Vitiation of tissue).

"अव्यायामाद्दिवास्वप्नान्मेद्यानां चातिभक्षणात् ।
मेदोवाहीनि दुष्यन्ति वारूण्याश्चातिसेवनात् ॥"
(च.वि.-५/१५)

Factors like Avyayama (no exercise), Diwaswapna (day sleep), excessive consumption of Medya Ahara (fatty diet) and Varuni (alcohol) leads to Medovaha Srotodushti (vitiation in channels of fatty tissue) causing a state of khavaigunya in the Meda Dhatu (fatty tissue).

Varuni can be correlated to beer which is a popular drink in today's culture. It is to be noted that beer has a high calorific value. Binging on beer also develops a characteristic central obesity which is popularly known as "beer belly". This also adds to the dyslipidemic effect of beer. Excessive alcohol consumption results in increase in plasma triglycerides.

On the basis of Samanya Vishesha Siddhanta (Principles of Similarity & Disimilarity) mentioned in Charak Samhita, the excessive consumption of similar substances i.e Dravyasamanya (Similar substance), similar qualities i.e Gunasamanya or similar action i.e Karmasamanya helps in the over production of the Dhatu (tissue).

When one or two or all three properties are similar, then such substances boost up the growth of the Dhatus (Tissues) which results as Dhatuvriddhi (Increase in tissue). Same way growth of Medo Dhatu (Fatty tissue) is observed by excessive consumption of –

1. Dravyasamanya (Similar substance): Medas (animal and plant fat).
2. Gunasamanya (similar qualities) :
   - Foods with Snigdha (oiliness), Guru(heavy) Guna like Ghrita (Ghee), Vasa (fat), Taila (oil), Milk, Mamsa (meat).
   - Foods and drugs of Sheeta Virya (Cold potency).
   - Substances with Madhura Rasa and Vipaka.
3. Karmasamanya (Similar action): Sedentary lifestyle, no exercise, day sleep, etc.

In hyperlipidaemia circulating lipids plays an important role. As these lipids can be well compared to Asthayi or Poshaka Medodhatu (unstable nutrient of fatty tissue); therefore it can be considered under Santarpanjanya Vikara (diseases of Overnutrition). Though there is no direct reference is found in the list of diseases described by Acharya Charak under the heading of Santarpanottha Vikaras (diseases of Overnutrition). Hence Nidanas (Etiology) of Santarpanotha

Vikaras (diseases of Overnutrition) can be well considered as Nidanas (Etiology) of hyperlipidaemia.

"संतर्पयति यः स्निग्धैर्मधुरैर्गुरूपिच्छिलैः ।

नवान्नैर्नवमद्यैश्च मांसैश्चानूपवारिजैः ।

गौरसैर्गौडिकैश्चान्नैः पैष्टिकैश्चातिमात्रशः ।

चेष्टाद्वेषी दिवास्वप्नशय्यासनसुखे रतः ॥"

(च.सु.-२३/३-४)

The above etiological factors can be broadly classified as Aharaja (Dietetics) and viharaja (Daily regime) Nidana (Etiology).

Aharaja Nidana (Dietetics etiology):

- Food qualities: Guru (heavy), Madhura (sweet), Sheeta (cold), Snigdha (oily), Shleshmala (mucus), Atipicchil (oversticky), Abhishyandi (slimy).

  The above qualities are present in Dravyas (substances) having a dominance of Prithvi (earth) and Apa (water) Mahabhuta (element). Due to similiar Bhautika (physical) composition the above substances are seen to cause a direct increase in the Kapha Dosha (phlegm) and Medo Dhatu (fatty tissue).
- Food items : Navanna(New grains), Navamadya(Newly prepared alcohol), Audaka rasa(Meat soup), Mamsa Sevana(Meat), Paya Vikara, Dadhi(Curd), Sarpi(Ghee), Ikshu Vikara(Sugarcane), Guda Vikara(Jaggery), Shali(Rice), Godhuma(Wheat), Masha(black gram), Varuni(Beer). The above stated foods like Navanna(New grains), Ikshu(Sugarcane), Guda vikara, Shali(Rice), Godhuma(Wheat), Masha(Black gram) are mainly seen to be rich sources of carbohydrates. Excess of ingested carbohydrates present in the foods may be easily converted to fats. These fats are more saturated and have a high melting point. Excess consumption of protein rich foods like milk and milk products may also lead to an increase in the body lipids. If the intake of dietary protein exceeds its tissue usage it is converted into triglycerides and stored in the body.

Procedural defect of eating: Atisampurna, Adhyashana(over eating), Vishamashana(irregular eating), Viruddhashana(unsuitable eating), Samashana, Atyambupana(Excessive water drinking), Bhojanottara Jalpana(Drinking water immediately after food) etc. Atisampurna or overeating results in excess storage of energy exceeding its utilization. Also excessive caloric consumption of any source of food with an associated weight gain may lead to hypertriglyceridaemia through VLDL (Verylow density lipoprotein) increase.

Factors like Adhyashana (over eating), Vishamashana (irregular eating) and Viruddhashana (unsuitable eating) subsequently lead to Ama(unriped substance) formation. Ama (unriped substance) results in Srotorodha (obstruction in channels) causing further pathogenesis of the disease.

Viharaja Nidana:

- Avyayama (No exercise)
- Avyavaya (No intercourse)
- Divaswapa (Day sleep)
- Asyasukha (Sedentary lifestyle)
- Swapnasukha (Over soundsleep)
- Bhojanottara Snana (Bath immediately after eating)
- Bhojanottara Nidra (sleep immediately after eating)etc.

All the above mentioned factors lead to lesser energy expenditure than input resulting in corpulence.

Manas Nidana(Mental Causes):

- Harshanityatva (Being always Happy)
- Achinatanam (Not taking Tension)
- Manasonivvrutti (Not being involved mentally in anything)
- Shaukhyam (Pleasure) are enumerated as the causative factors by Acharya Charaka which is conducive to Atisthaulya (Excessive Obesity).

2. **Adrishtavashat :**

This pertains to factors mainly the hereditary or genetic factors which cannot be seen or assessed directly. These are mainly due to defects in the either the Shukra(Sperm) or Shonita

(Ovum) or both which are transmitted in the progeny. All the Acharyas have unanimously included genetic defects as a cause of Sthaulya (Obesity) and allied disorders like Prameha (Diabetes) etc. Acharya Charaka has also stated Beejadosha (defect in sperm & ovum) in as one of the etiological factors of Atisthaulya (Excessive Obesity). These genetic factors lead to development of a state of khavaigunya in the Medo Dhatu (fatty tissue) which making it susceptible for the action of vitiated Doshas.

Various genetic and hereditary factors are known to be responsible for causing Hyperlipidaemia which can also be termed as primary Hyperlipidaemia can be studied under the broad umbrella of "Beejadosha" (defect in sperm & ovum).

3. Medosavrita Margatvat(Obstruction in path of fat):

Commentator Dalhana has quoted that Vata Vikaras (Diseasesof air) or disorders of Vata occur due to Avarana (covering) of the Marga (path) by Medo Dhatu (fatty tissue). This refers to secondary conditions leading to Hyperlipidaemia like diabetes mellitus, hypothyroidism etc where a significant role is played by Vata in the pathogenesis. The normal Gati (movement) of Vata Dosha (air) gets obstructed due to excess of Medo Dhatu (fatty tissue) which thus gets vitiated causing further pathogenesis. These factors causing secondary Hyperlipidaemia can also be called as Nidanarthakari Roga since one disease serves as the etiological factor of the other.

"तदतिस्थौल्यमतिसम्पूरणाद् गुरुमधुरशीतस्निग्धोपयोगाद्
व्यायामादव्यवायाद्दिवास्वप्नाद्हर्षनित्यत्वादचिन्तनाद्बीजस्वभावाच्चोपजायते ।"

(च.सु.-२१/४)

The etiological factors described in the ayurvedic texts can be classified into 3 groups –

1. Ahara paraka hetu (Dietary causes)
2. Vihara paraka hetu (Physical causes)
3. Manasika hetu (psychological causes)
4. Other hetu (Causes)

1. Ahara Paraka Hetu (Dietary causes) –

➢ Guru Ati Sevan (Excessive intake of heavy food) – The Guru Ahara (heavy food) due to its Guru Paki (heavy transformation) and Sheeta virya (cold potency) property takes time to digest. It also affects Agni (metabolic fire) and as a result in increase of Kapha Dosha (phlegm) which further enrich Dushya Meda (Vitiated fat) .

- Madhura Ati Sevan (Excessive intake of sweet food) – The Madhura Rasa Pradhan diets usually have Sheeta (cold), Guru (heavy), Snigdha (oily) and Parthiva apya(earth water) property, such as Ghee, Payas, sugarcane products, banana, etc.
- Sheetahara Sevan (Intake of cold food) – Sheetahara (cold) usually have Parthivapya and Vayavya (earthwater & air) property. Due to the opposite of Ushna Guna (hot property) it produces the obstruction in channels and hampers the normal functions of the body in the manner increased Kapha Dosha (Phlegm) increases the Medo Dhatu (fatty tissue).
- Shlesma Bahula Ahara (excessive food containing phlegm)– Due to continuous intake of slesma bahula Ahara, the similar Dhatus (tissue) especially Meda Dhatu(fatty tissue) is being increased by the principal of Samanya Vriddhi Karanam (causes of increase of similarity).
- Atibhojana (Excessive eating)– Excessive eating may aggravate all the Doshas (bodily humor) and affect the Pachakagni (digestive fire) leading to delayed and improper digestion. As a result Amarasa (unriped/immature fluid) is formed and it spreads over whole of the body.
- Adhyashana (over eating)– Adhyasana (over eating) again disturbs the normal physiological state of Jatharagni (digestive fire) so that improper digestion of food take place and formation of Ama (unriped substance) is resulted. This Ama (unriped substance) further mixes with Kapha (phlegm) and Medo Dhatu (fatty tissue) due to similar properties so that Medo Dhatu Dusti (vitiation of fatty tissue) results.
- Pistanna Ati Sevan (excessive eating of grained food)- These types of foods are difficult to digest and aggravate the kapha Dosha (phlegm). Due to difficulty in digestion of these foods they produces Ama (unriped substance) by affecting the Pachakagni (digestive fire) as a result the Dhatwagni (tissue fire) especially Medo Dhatwagni (fatty tissue fire) becomes Manda (slow) so that Sama Medo Dhatu results and leads to Medo Dhatu Dusti (vitiation of fatty tissue).

2. Vihara Paraka Hetu (Physical causes) -

- Avyayama (No exercise) - Lack of exercise or sedentary life style will leads to Ama Ama (unriped substance) formation at various levels. This Ama Ama (unriped substance) further enriches the Sama Meda Ama (unriped fat) and ultimately Medo Dhatu Dusti (vitiation of fatty tissue) results.

- Avyavaya (No intercourse) – Due to lack of sexual indulgence the Shukra Dhatu (sperm) increases and it may produce Srotorodha (obstruction in channels) if it is prolonged with continuous intake of Santarpana (overnutritious) diet, it leads to increase of Medo Dhatu (fatty tissue).
- Diwaswapna (Day sleep)– Day time sleep increases the Kapha Dosha (phlegm). If the day sleep is practiced continuously then it obstructs the channels by increasing the Kapha Dosha (phlegm), as a result it causes the Medo Dhatu Dusti (vitiation of fatty tissue).

3. Mansika Hetu (Psycological factors) –

- Achintana (No thinking/worry) – Chintana means mental exercise or work. Acharya Charaka has clearly mentioned Snehana (oiling) therapy for those regularly do mental work in excess because Chintana (thinking) leads to aggravation of Vata Dosha (air). Whereas Achintana (no thinking) increases Kapha Dosha (phlegm) and increased Kapha Dosha (phlegm) due to the similar properties enriches Medo Dhatu (fatty tissue) also.
- Nitya Harsa (always joyful) – Means continuously joy. The continuous joy leads to increase of the bodily tissue (Dhatu). If one takes the nourishing diet daily with joy then it leads to increase in the Kapha Dosha (phlegm) and likewise Dhatu (tissue) also.

4. Other Hetu(Causes)-

"बीजस्वभावादिति स्थूल मातापितृजन्यत्वात् ।
संश्राति स्थूलस्य साधारणादव्याहार भूरिमेदो जन्माहतस्यहीत्यादि ।" (चक्रपाणि टिका) च.सु.-२१/४)

Other Hetu (causes) includes Beeja Swabhava (defect in cells). Acharyas have mentioned the Beeja Swabhavaja (defect in cells) as the causative factor of Sthaulya (obesity). Here it refers genetic factors responsible for some forms of Hyperlipidaemia.

Beejadoshaja Nidanas (causes of cellular defect):

This pertains to factors mainly the heredity or genetic factors which cannot be seen or assessed directly. These are mainly due to defects in the either the Shukra (sperm) or Shonita (ovum) or both which are transmitted in the progeny. All the Acharyas have unanimously included genetic defects as a cause of Sthaulya (obesity) and allied disorders like Prameha (Diabetic) etc. Acharya Charaka has also stated Beejadosha (defect in cells) as one of the etiological factors of

Atisthaulya (obesity). These genetic factors lead to development of a state of Khavaigunya in the Medodhatu (fatty tissue) which making it susceptible for the action of vitiated Doshas (bodily humor). Various genetic and heredity factors are known to be responsible for causing Hyperlipidemia which can also be termed as Primary Hyperlipidaemia can be studied under the broad umbrella of Beejadosha (defect in cells).

5.6 Purvaroopa (Prodromal Symptoms) And Rupa (Clinical Manifestations):

Purvaroopa (Prodromal Symptoms)

The premonitory symptoms of the disease Hyperlipidaemia or Medo Dhatu Dusti (Vitiation in fatty tissue) are not described in the Ayurvedic text but due to its similarity with Kapha Dosha (phlegm) Aggravation, the initial symptoms of Kapha Vriddhi (increase in phlegm) like Aruchi (anorexia), Alasya (laziness), Gaurav (heaviness), Nidra (sleep), Tandra (lethargy), etc may be considered as the Poorvarupa (prodromal) of Medo Dhatu Dusti (vitiation of fatty tissue). The disease Hyperlipidaemia is not preceded by any premonitory signs and symptoms. Thus, the Avyakta Lakshanas(Unmanifested symptoms) of Hyperlipidaemia can be taken as its Purvarupa (prodromal).

Rupa (Clinical Manifestations):

The signs and symptoms of the disease as seen on the body are Avyakta(Unmanifest) or Alpavyakta(less manifest). The diagnosis of the disease is mainly done by assessing the Lipid Profile.

5.7 Samprapti (Pathogenesis):

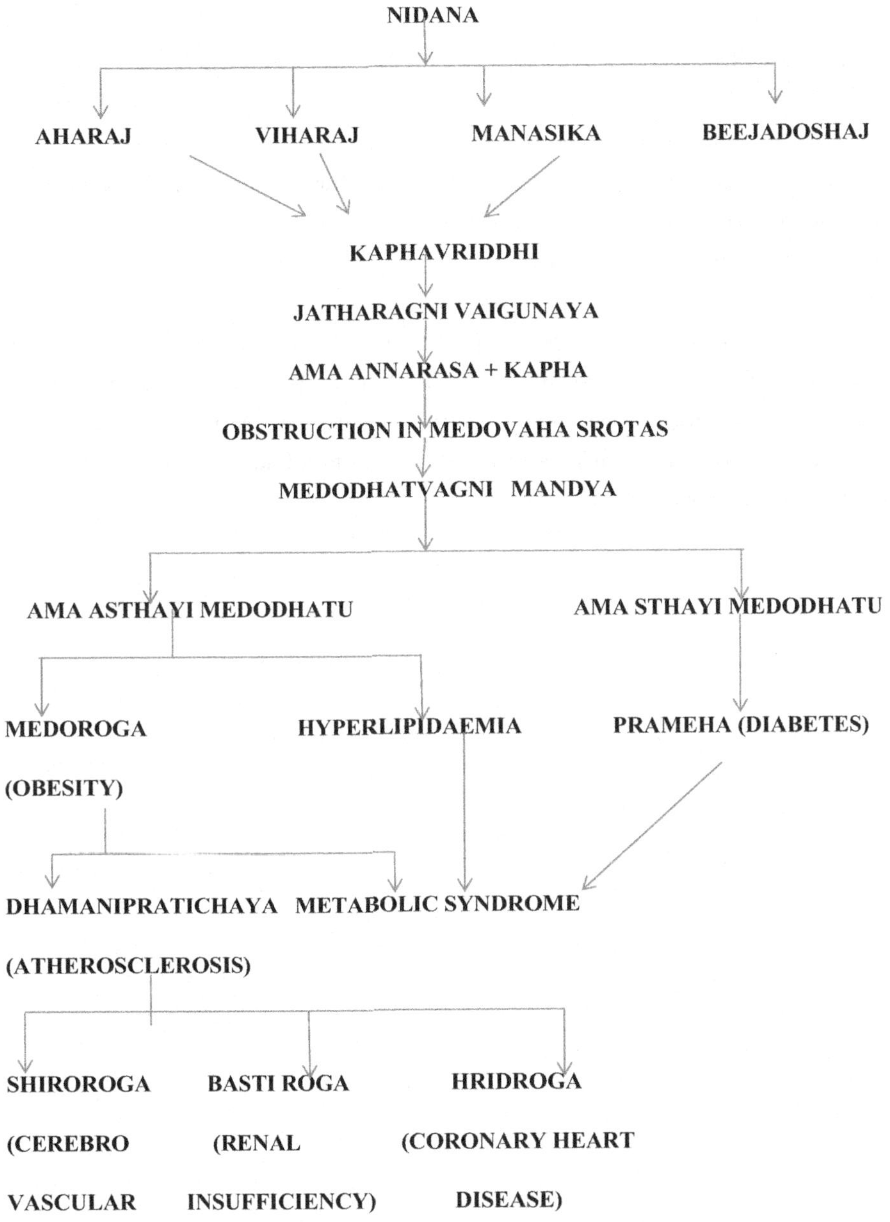

5.8 Upadrava (Complications):

When Dusta Meda (unripened/ improperly formed) is increased extensively it give rise to various clinical manifestation known as Medoroga (Disease of fat). Medoroga (Disease of fat) and Medodosha (defects in fat) have been described to the synonyms of each other. Literally it means disease where Medodhatu (fatty tissue) is involved. But Adhamalla, commentator of Atankadarpana on Sharangdhara has tried to distinguish two type of Medoroga.

1. Medodusti (Hyperlipidaemia / Dyslipidaemia)
2. Sthaulya (Adiposity)

In Medodusti condition Apachita (undigested) or Samameda(Unriped fat) acts as an etiological factor in the production of other disease for example in Hridroga (heart disease) due to Medodusti (Hyperlipidaemia) Samameda(Unriped fat) accumulates in Hridayagata Dhamnis (arteries of heart) a condition known as Dhamani pratichaya (Atherosclerosis) which leads to obstruction of vessels and ultimately Hridroga (heart disease) develop.

5.9 Ayurvedic Management Of Hyperlipidaemia :

"संशोधनं संशमनं निदानस्य च वर्जनम् ।
एतावद् भिषजा कार्यं रोगे रोगे यथाविधि ॥"
(च. वि.-७/३०)

The treatment of Hyperlipidaemia i.e - Asthayi Medodhatu Vriddhi (unstable increase of fatty tissue) can be elaborated by using Ayurvedic view.

General principle of Management disorder is divided into three parts.

1. Nidanaparivarjana (Avoiding the cause)
2. Samshodhana (Purification)
3. Samshamana (Palliative care)
4. Pathya and Apathya(Do's and dont's)

1. **Nidanaparivarjana** (Avoiding the cause): Nidana (etiology) such as Kapha (phlegm) provocating Medovahasrotas (Fatty tissue channels) vitiating, Medovriddhikara Ahara & Vihara (Dietetics and daily regime causing increase of fat) should be avoided strictly

2. **Samshodhana (Purification):**
   Bahya Shodhana (external purification) :

"उद्वर्तनं कफहरं मेदसः प्रविलापनम ।
स्थिरीकरणम् अङ्गानां त्वक्प्रसादकरं परं ॥"
(अ. हृ . सु - २/१५)

"वातघ्नान्यन्नपानानि श्लेष्ममेदोहरानि च ।
रुक्षोष्णा बस्तयस्तीक्ष्णा रूक्षाण्युद्वर्तनानि च | (च. सु.२१/२१)

For Bahya Shodhana (external purification) Udvartana (rubbing of dry herbal powder over body) has been mentioned in charak samhita. In Ashtanga Hridaya its property likes, Kaphahara (phlegm alleviating), Medas Pravilayana (dissolution of fat), Sthirikaranam Anganam(stabilization in body) etc. is mentioned. It helps in removing foetid odour, restricts the excess sweating and alleviates the aggravated Doshas (bodily humor).

Some Udvartana Dravyas (Rubbing Of Dry Herbal Powder Over Body) And Their Probable Mode Of Action :

1. Triphala churna
2. Kulatha churna
3. Vidanga churna
4. Haridra churna
5. Vacha churna
6. Shilajatu churna
7. Musta churna

having properties to alleviate stagnant kapha (phlegm) , meda (fat) , ama (undigested food) - due to their ushna virya (hot potency) and katu vipak (pungent endproduct). Laghu(light) , ruksha (dry) , suksma (subtle) guna (property)causes excess kleda shoshan (moisture absorption).

Abhyantara Samshodhana (Internal Purification):

"शस्तमुल्लेखनं तत्र विरेको रक्तमोक्षणम् ।
व्यायामश्चोपवासश्च धूमश्च स्वेदनानि च ॥
सक्षौद्रश्चाभयाप्राशः प्रायो रुक्षान्नसेवनम् ।
चूर्णप्रदेहा ये चोक्ताः कण्डूकोठविनाशनाः ॥"
(च. सू. २३/ ८-९)

Being a syndromic entity Samshodhana (purifactory) therapy is highly recommended for Hyperlipidaemia. Charaka has mentioned Vamana (emesis), Virechana (purgation), Raktamokshana (blood letting) for Santarpanottha Vikaras (diseases of overnutrition) which can be used for treating Hyperlipidaemia. He also suggested Ruksha (dry), Tikshna (strong) & Ushna basti (hot enema) for management of Sthaulya (obesity) which can be suitable for Hyperlipidaemia.

Samshamana (Palliative):

Among Shadupakramas, Langhana(fasting) & Rukshana (drying) can be administered for Samshamana (palliative) purpose. All the seven ways of Langhana (fasting) can be applied to the patient of Hyperlipidaemia according to Rogi-Roga Bala (patient-disease strength).

1. Deepana(Augmentation)
2. Pachana(Digestion)
3. Vyayama(Exercise)

4. Marutasevana(Intake of air)
5. Atapasevana(Intake of heat)
6. Kshut-Nigraha(Hunger control)
7. Trishnanigraha(Thirst control)

Some Hypolipidaemic Formulations considered as lipid regulating mentioned in Ayurveda:

1. Arogyavardhini Vati
2. Navak Guggula
3. Arjuna Vati
4. Tab Abana
5. Prabhakar Vati
6. Triphala Guggula
7. Lasunadi Guggula

Table No: 10 Pathya and Apathya(Do's and Don'ts):

PATHYA	APATHYA
Moonga,	Adhyashana
Yava,	Atibhojana
Madhu,	Vishamabhojana
Paravala,	Virudhabhojana
Anara,	Atyambupana
Takra,	Madhura- Snigdha-Pistanna Sevana
Shunthi,	Dadhi
Ardraka,	Udada
Lahasuna,	Chavala
Amalaki,	Mamsa
Soya,	Fish,
Haritaki,	Egg yolk
Ushna Jala,	Butter
Sarshapa taila	Vegadharana
Vyayama	Diwaswapa etc.
Sharama	
Langhana	

CHAPTER 6 - CLINICAL CASE PRESENTATION:

RESEARCH WORK

CLINICAL EVALUATION OF EFFICACY OF RASARAKTA PACHAK GHANAVATI IN HYPERLIPIDAEMIA (RASAGAT SNEHA VRIDDHI)

6.1 Introduction Of Study:

The growing challenges of modernization have resulted in human beings readjusting their customary behavior by modifying their dietary and lifestyle preferences. Fast or junk foods, less or lack of exercise, psychological stress, etc. are some of the factors which are adversely impacting the lifestyle of man in the 21st century. Diet rich with saturated or trans fats along with physical inactivity is also considered as major cause for hyperlipidaemia. This has resulted in a discrepancy between external environment and man's internal body mechanism which leads to a multitude of diseases, mainly due to impaired metabolism, these are referred to as lifestyle diseases and Hyperlipidemia is one such disorder.

Hyperlipidemia is a term used to denote increased levels of Total Cholesterol, Triglycerides (TGs), or both i.e. Cholesterol and Triglycerides. Hyperlipidaemia, due to the modifications of serum/plasma lipid profile, is consider as a major cause of cardiac disorders, such as coronary artery disease (CAD) and other diseases such as ischaemic cerebrovascular disease, and peripheral vascular disease. Coronary artery disease (CAD) is considered as one of the most common cause of mortality and morbidity in both developed and developing countries.

Herbs have been used in medical treatment since the beginning of civilization and have become a mainstay of human pharmacotherapy. Based on this, many research works were carried out in evaluating the lipid lowering effects of plants and from the reports on their potential effectiveness, it is assumed that botanicals have a major role to play in management of hyperlipidemia.

Now a days synthetic drugs have been associated with number of side effects but herbal medicines have lipid lowering and antioxidant activity and probably without any major side effects. Medicinal plants have been considered as healthy source of life for all peoples due to its rich therapeutic properties and being 100% natural.

There is no direct reference in Ayurved of a particular disease entity that can be correlated with hyperlipidemia. The study of Ayurveda texts bears certain unclear concepts or reference relating to an increase in amount of Rasagat Sneha (circulating body lipids), yet the literal meaning of hyperlipidemia is not found to be specifically stated anywhere. The lipids which are elevated can be correlated to excess of Sneha (oil), Meda dhatu(fatty tissue), Samarasa due to the similarity in their properties. A detailed study of hyperlipidaemia reveals its resemblance to Asthayi Medo Dhatu Vriddhi (increase in unstable fatty tissue). Various scholars of Ayurveda made attempts to co–relate it to Rasagat Sneha Vriddhi, Raktagat Sneha Vriddhi, Rasaraktagat Sneha Vriddhi, Medoroga, Medo Vriddhi, Sama Medo Dhatu, Sthaulya, etc. By considering all the situations it can be presumed that the pathology is related to Kapha dosha (phlegm) increasing aetiological factors i.e. – Santarpana aahara, vihara (over nutritious diet & daily regime), which includes sedentary life style, food consisting high calories, very less or lack of exercise which leads to morbidity of Kapha dosha (phlegm) and Medo dhatu (fatty tissue) and causes Santarpanjanya vyadhi (Diseases due to over nutrition).

This kind of Medodhatu vruddhi (increase in fatty tissue) which is Aama(unriped/ undigested) in nature hence it is retained in the body for a longer time and causes further complications. It can be implicit that the pathology is related to Kapha (phlegm) vitiation hetu (etiology) i.e. – Santarpana aahara, vihara, which includes sedentary lifestyle, excessive snigdha (fatty) food intake, lack of exercise, etc impairs digestion (agnimandya) which finally leads to excess of Kapha dosha and Medo dhatu. Due to impaired Meda dhatu agni, excessive Kapha and Meda get accumulated in different srotas. Aparipakva Kapha–Meda in Rasaraktavaha Srotas causes obstruction to Vata dosha and Rakta, which at last ends up in disease manifestation according to the site of infirmity.

Concept of Agni (metabolic fire) in Ayurveda defines collectively all bodily metabolic actions. Low Agni(metabolic fire) is the cause for formation of Aama (unriped/undigested food), which can obstruct the metabolic pathways and causing diseases. Correction of Agni (metabolic fire) is the principle of treatment for increased lipid levels. An Ayurvedic approach to hyperlipidaemia involves methods to increase power of Agni (metabolic fire) and to digest the Aama (unriped/undigested food). Hence, this study was carried out to evaluate clinically the efficacy of Rasarakta Pachak Ghanavati in Hyperlipidaemia

6.2 Aim And Objectives Of Study:

Aim :-

To evaluate the efficacy of Rasarakta Pachak Ghanavati in Hyperlipidaemia.

Objectives –

1. To study the Hyperlipidaemia condition in detail.
2. To study present day dietary habits and lifestyle as a causative factor for hyperlipidaemia.
3. To study the concept and role of Agnideepan(Augmentation of metabolic fire) and Amapachan(Digestion of Undigested food) in the management of hyperlipidaemia.

6.3 Materials And Methodology:

After approval from Institutional Ethics Committee, 60 patients of hyperlipidaemia, fulfilling inclusion criteria and willing to give written informed consent were selected randomly from OPD/IPD.

Group A received the Rasarakta Pachak Ghanavati which is a polyherbal combination of Kalinga/Indrayava (Holarhhena antidysentrica), Patola (Tricosanthes dioica), Katuka (Pichrorhiza kurroa), Sariva (Hemedismus indicus), Musta (Cyperus rotundus), Patha (Cissampelos pareira) in equal quantity as mentioned in Charak Samhita Chikitsasthan Jwara Chapter 3/200.

Group B patients were treated with Atorvastatin (Lipitor) which is a member of the drug class known as statins used for lowering cholesterol.

Table 8: Method of drug administration and study design

	Group A (Trial Group)	**Group B (Control Group)**
Drug	Rasarakta Pachak Ghanavati	Tab Atorvastatin
Dose	500mg 2 tab twice in a day	10 mg 1 tab once in a day
Kala	Vyanodana(after meal)	After meal
Route	Oral	Oral
Anupan	Ushnodak (Tepid water)	Water
Duration	30 days	30 days
Follow up	0, 30th day	0, 30th day

6.4 Criteria For Selection Of Patient:

Inclusion Criteria:

1. Age limit from 30 to 60 years.
2. Patient of either sex of Hyperlipidaemia.
3. Newly detected or known case of Hyperlipidemia.
4. Range of lipid- Sr.TotalCholesterol–>200mg/dl; Sr.Triglycerides–>150md/dl; Sr.HDL-Cholesterol-<40mg/dl; Sr.LDL-Cholesterol->130mg/dl.

Exclusion Criteria:

1. Patient below the age of 30 and above 60 years.
2. Pregnant women and lactating mother.
3. Chronic infection/illness like TB, HIV, Cancer, hypertension, Diabetes mellitus, renal diseases, coronary heart diseases.
4. Known case of psychological disorders like anxiety, depression were excluded.

Criteria for assessment:

Diagnostic and objective parameters for assessment was as per American Journal of Lifestyle Medicine and accordingly scoring pattern was set. Patient was diagnosed based on lipid profile.

6.5 Results:

Table 9: Group A (Trial group) Before and After Treatment Comparison

	Mean	SD	Mean difference	SD Difference	% Improvement	Paired T test	P value
Sr.C (D0)	233.53	36.653	29.167	39.158	90%	4.080	0.0001
Sr.C (D30)	204.37	44.945					
Sr.TG (D0)	157.83	96.930	-0.633	99.426	50%	-.035	0.972
Sr.TG (D30)	158.47	112.88					
Sr.HDL-C (D0)	35.60	10.091	0.000	14.096	53.33%	.000	1.000
Sr.HDL-C (D30)	35.60	14.148					
Sr.LDL-C (D0)	164.33	38.219	24.233	32.685	76.66%	4.061	0.0001
Sr.LDL-C (D30)	140.10	41.156					

Graph 1: Test of Significance for Group A

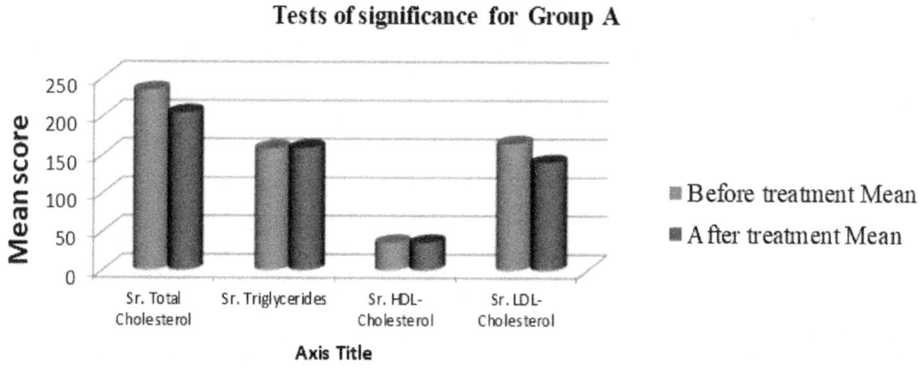

Table 10: Group B (Control group) before and after treatment comparison

	Mean	SD	Range	Median	% Improvement	Wilcoxon Signed Ranks Test value	P value
Sr.C (D0)	216.33	37.716	147-360	212.50	96.66%	-4.762	0.0001
Sr.C (D30)	168.50	38.637	101-290	172.00			
Sr.TG (D0)	145.70	71.849	50-294	120.50	76.66%	-2.900	0.004
Sr.TG (D30)	120.03	56.835	48-267	105.00			
Sr.HDL-C (D0)	37.97	11.421	18-60	37.50	80%	-2.533	0.011
Sr.HDL-C (D30)	33.37	7.933	21-54	31.00			
Sr.LDL-C (D0)	147.80	40.850	66-293	148.50	90%	-4.628	0.0001
Sr.LDL-C (D30)	111.00	33.411	46-205	110.00			

Graph 2: Test of Significance for Group B

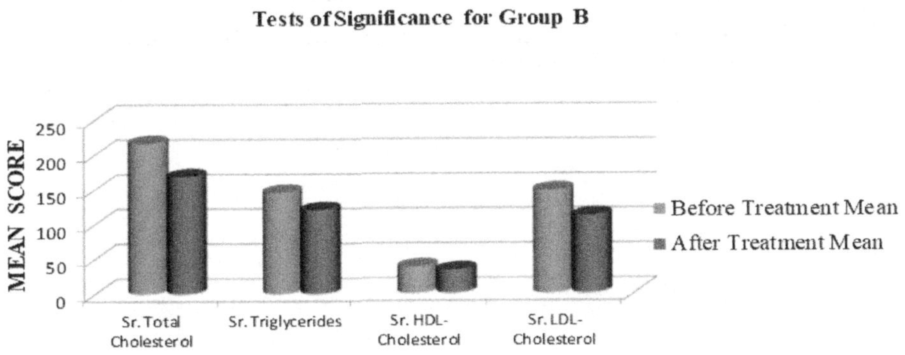

Table 11: Percentage wise overall improvement in Group A and Group B:

Lipid profile	Group A %Relief	Group B %Relief
Serum Cholesterol	90%	96.66%
Serum Triglycerides	50%	76.66%
Serum HDL-Cholesterol	53.33%	80%
Serum LDL-Cholesterol	76.66%	90%

<u>Graph 3: Percentage wise overall improvement in Group A and Group B</u>

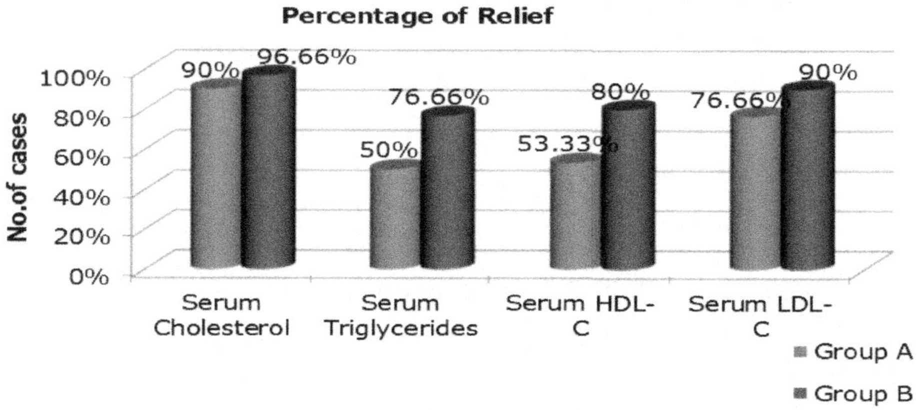

6.6 Discussion:

Considering the etiopathogenesis of Hyperlipidaemia it can be considered as a disease due to excess nutrition (Santarpanjanya Vikara). Being a metabolic syndrome there lies a definite relation between pathophysiology of Hyperlipidaemia with Agnivaigunya (low digestive fire) at different levels starting from Jatharagni (digestive fire) up to Dhatvagni (tissue fire). In Charak Samhita it is mentioned Atisthaulya (obesity) as one of the Kaphaja Nanatmaja Vikara (diseases due to vitiation of Kapha dosha) in the Chapter Maharoga(Severe Diseases) and is later elaborated upon in the subsequent Ashtau Ninditiya Adhyaya (eight undesired persons). On further observation it is evident that Atisthaulya (obesity) is physiology predominant disorder which eventually gets converted into a pathological state.

Acharya Charaka has stated the main vitiated Dosha (bodily humor) responsible for the pathogenesis in Prameha (Diabetic) as Bahu Drava Shleshma (excess Kapha) and the main vitiated Dushya (tissue) as—Bahu Abaddha Medas or Medas (excess fat tissue) which is greater in quantity but is free in circulation. This Abaddha Medas (unbined fat) or Asthayi Medo dhatu (Unstable fatty tissue) can be compared to lipoproteins which are seen to increase diabetes mellitus.

Now day's synthetic drugs have been associated with number of side effects. But herbal medicines have lipid lowering and antioxidant activity, probably without any major side effects. Recently herbal hypolipidemics have gained importance to fill the lacunae created by the allopathic drugs. Modern medicine i.e., statins and fibrates are established drugs available for Hyperlipidaemia, which are useful but if someone is taking these medicines for a longer duration shows some side effects i.e., diarrhoea, dizziness, constipation, flatulence, stomach upset, muscle pain and must be taken throughout life.

As per Ayurvedic view if such modern medicines taken for long duration, it decreases Sneha(oiliness) present in body and causes vitiation of Vata(air). Hence for treating hyperlipidaemia cases, Rasarakta Pachak Ghanavati with Ushnodak (tepid water) has been chosen.

In Charak Samhita it is mentioned that Rasarakta Pachak Yoga is to be given in the form of kwath (Decoction), but for the palatability and convenience of the patient and to increase the potency of medicine Ghanavati (extract in tablet form) is prepared and named as Rasarakta Pachak GhanaVati.

Pharmacological effect of Rasarakta Pachak Ghanavati:

Rasarakta Pachak Ghanavati pacifies all the three doshas (TridoshaShamaka) but especially pacifies vitiation of Kapha dosha which is dominant in the pathogenesis of Hyperlipidaemia as well as depletes the excessively produced Rasa (plasma), Mamsa(Muscle), Meda(Fat), Vasa(Fatty deposits), Sweda (Sweating), and Kleda which are all similar in attributes to Kapha dosha. Thus, it is known to act against the vitiated kapha (Kaphapradhan) pathogenesis of Hyperlipidaemia. The drugs like Patha (Cissampelospariera), Sariva (Hemedismus indicus), Musta (Cyperusrotundus) does Mutravirechana(Diuresis) and take out excessive Kleda(Moisture), whereas Musta (Cyperusrotundus), Patola (Tricosanthesdioica), Patha (Cissampelospariera), Katuka (Pichrorhizakurroa), Kalinga (Holarhhena antidysentrica) increases the digestive fire leading to proper formation of the Rasadi Dhatu (plasma etc tissues). Patola (Tricosanthesdioica) and Katuka (Pichrorhizakurroa) have purgative action which causes Anulomana of Vayu (Download movement of vayu) and breaks the Vata pradhana (air dominant) Samprapti (pathogenesis).

Drugs like Musta (Cyperusrotundus), Patola (Tricosanthesdioica), Patha (Cissampelospariera), Katuka (Pichrorhizakurroa), having Pachan (Digestive) property digest the Aama Dosha (Undigested food) present at the Jatharagni (Digestive fire) level as well as the Medodhatvagni (Fatty tissue) level. Drugs like Katuka (Pichrorhizakurroa) and Musta (Cyperusrotundus) by doing lekhan (Scrapping) removes excess kleda (Moisture), Meda (Fat) from the Srotas (Channels).

Pharmacological effect of Tab Atorvastatin:

Atorvastatin are potent inhibitors of the rate liming enzyme involved in sterol synthesis, HMG-CoA reductase. It is a reversible competitor of the 3-hydroxy 3-methyl glutaryl coenzyme A reductase (HMGCoA). It competitively inhibits HMG coenzyme a reductase, which is involved in the rate limiting step of cholesterol biosynthesis in the liver. It acts by binding to the critical catalytic site of the enzyme. Hence the blockage of the enzyme later reduces de novo cholesterol production, increasing expression of LDL lipoprotein receptors on hepatocytes. This increases LDL uptake the hepatocytes, decreasing the amount of LDL Cholesterol in the blood. Also, helpful to reduce levels of triglycerides and slightly increases levels of HDL Cholesterol. Thus, mechanism of action was found to inhibit liver cholesterol synthesis by acting on HMGCoA, decreased LDL and increased

HDL level, this causes increase in lipolytic activity in liver and heart, increases excretion of bile acids and cholesterol in faces.

The study of effect of Rasarakta Pachak Ghanavati and Tab Atorvastatin in hyperlipidaemia was done on 60 patients. Clinical data obtained from the study was entered in Microsoft excel and analysed using SPSS20 software to check any difference between effect of drug (Group A and B) on lipid profile. Test of normality was applied to check normal distribution of data. For normally distributed data T test was applied and for not normally distributed data Wilcoxon signed rank test was applied, Data was statistically analysed and percentage of improvement, mean value, P value were calculated by using "t" test and "Wilcoxon signed rank test" and presented in observations and results were discussed on Demographic Analysis, clinical effect of drug on objective parameters of lipid profile, probable mechanism of action of drug and total effect of therapy.

RESULT:

Total effect of therapy:

Group A (Rasarakta Pachak Ghanavati) showed marked improvement on Serum Cholesterol and Serum LDL – Cholesterol and moderate improvement on Serum Triglycerides and Serum HDL – Cholesterol parameters of lipid Profile. Whereas in Group B (Tab Atorvastatin) showed marked improvement on all the parameters of lipid profile.

In Group A (Rasarakta Pachak Ghanavati) statistically marked improvement was observed on Serum Cholesterol (90%) and LDL – C(76.66%) and moderate improvement observed on Sr. TG(50%) and Sr. HDL –C(53.33%). This shows that Rasarakta Pachak Ghanavati is quite better effective in Hyperlipidaemia. Whereas in Group B (Tab Atorvastatin) statistically marked improvement was observed on all the four parameters of lipid profile i.e. – Sr. Cholesterol (96.66%) Sr. TG (76.66%) and Sr. HDL –C (80%) Sr. LDL – C (90%).

6.7 Conclusion:

Hyperlipidemia is one of the major risk factors which is related with Atherosclerosis and atherosclerosis induced conditions like coronary artery disease (CAD). Hypolipidemic drugs are those, which lower the level of lipids and lipoproteins in blood. A rise in LDL may cause deposition of cholesterol in the arteries and aorta and hence it is a direct risk factor for coronary heart disease.

Wide range of drugs i.e. statins, fibrates, resins, etc., which are quite effective in normalizing the lipid levels gives only symptomatic relief for months or years, also by taking these medicines for a longer duration shows some side effects i.e. diarrhoea, dizziness, headache, constipation, flatulence, stomach upset, myalgia, increase level of serum transaminase which can further leads to liver damage, etc. and also have to take throughout life.

As per Ayurveda view if such modern medicines taken for longer duration it decreases Sneha(Oiliness) present in the body and causes vitiation of Vata(Air). The symptoms of Hyperlipidaemia described in modern text shows resemblance with the Aam(Unriped/Undigestedmaterial), and with Rasa Dushti(Vitiation in plasma), Rakta dushti Vitiation in plasma),, and Medodushti Janya (Causing vitiation in Fat) symptoms. Correction of Agni(Metabolic fire) is the basic treatment for increased lipid levels.

An Ayurveda approach to Hyperlipidemia involves methods to increase power of Agni(Metabolic fire) and to digest the Ama(Unriped/Undigestedmaterial). Drugs having properties like Dipana(Augmenting), Amapachana(Digestive), Kapha-Meda Shamana (Palliation of Phlegm-Fat), Yakrituttejaka(Liver stimulating), Srotoshodhaka(Purificatory of channels and Lekhana(Scraping) which forcefully clears the accumulated Ama(Unriped/Undigestedmaterial) in the Srotas (Channels) can be used.

Hyperlipidaemia can be treated on the principles of Apatarpan chikitsa (reduction therapy) mentioned in Ayurveda. Rasarakta Pachak Ghanavati provided better results on lipid profile by showing marked reduction especially on Serum Cholesterol and Serum LDL- Cholesterol which was well appreciated within one month duration.

During study no adverse effects of Rasarakta Pachak Ghanavati was noted. As study was of limited duration but if Rasarakta Pachak Ghanavati continued for longer duration, it will be more effective in Hyperlipidaemia.

Thus, it can be concluded that Rasarakta Pachak Ghanavati is effective in lipid profile and can be used for the treatment of Hyperlipidaemia as a safest and effective drug for long term duration without any side effects.

REFERENCES

1. Human Physiology, Dr. C. C. Chatterjee, Medical Allied Agency, tenth edition 1997.
2. Dr. V Satyanarayana, U.Chakrapani, Text Book of Biochemistry, Books And Allied (P) Ltd. Edition: Reprint 2009.
3. K.Sembulingam, Prema Sembulinga, Essentials of Medical Physiology, Jaypee Brothers Medical Publishers (P) LTD NewDelhi, Edition: 6th 2013.
4. Kasper Hauser, Braunwald Longo, Frauci Jameson, Harrison's Principles of Internal Medicine (Vol II), Edition: 16th edition.
5. Kaviraja Ambikadutta Shastri, Foreword by Dr. Pranajivana Mehta, Sushruta Samhita of Maharshi Sushruta (part I), edited with Ayurveda Tattva Sandipika, Chaukhambha Sanskrit Sansthan Varanasi, Reprinted – 2010.
6. C.Dwarkanath, Digestion & Metabolism in Ayurveda, Chaukhambha Krishnadas Academy Varanasi, Edition: Reprint 2010.
7. Dr.Siddharth N. Shah, API Text book of Medicine (vol II), Edition- 8th edition reprint 2009.
8. K.D Tripathi , Essentials of Medical Pharmacology, , Jaypee Brothers Medical Publishers (P) LTD, Edition: 6th reprint 2010.
9. Acharya Vidyadhar Shukla, Prof. Ravi Dutt Tripathi ,Charak samhita of Agnivesha (Volume I) edited with 'Vaidyamanorama' Hindi Commentary,Chaukhamba Sanskrit Pratishthan Delhi, Reprinted – 2009.
10. Sushrut samhita, edited by P. V. Sharma, vol.1,3rd edition, Chaukhamba oriental, Varanasi, Sutra sthan, Dalhan commentary on cha.5/5, 2007.
11. Vaidya V.M.Gogte, Ayurvedic Pharmacology and Therapeutic uses of Medicinal Plants Dravyaguna Vignyan, Chaukhambha Publication New Delhi, Edition: Reprint 2012.
12. Singh R. H.; The holistic principles of Ayurveda medicine; Delhi: Chaukhamba Sanskrit pratishthan; 2003.
13. Manjiri Arun Nadkarni et al Randomized placebo-controlled trial of Mustadi Ghanavati in hyperlipidemia Ayu. 2010 Jul;31(3):287-93. doi: 10.4103/0974-8520.77150.
14. Brahmanand Tripathi, Astanga Hridaya, Sutra sthan, chapter 2, verse no.15, Edition Reprint 2017, Vol no 1, Delhi Chaukhamba Sanskrit Pratishthan.

Publisher: Eliva Press Global Ltd

Email: info@elivapress.com

Made in United States
North Haven, CT
04 November 2026

21772728R00055